Embedding Evidence-Based Practice in Speech and Language Therapy

Embedding Evidence-Based Practice in Speech and Language Therapy: International Examples

Edited by

Hazel Roddam
Principal Lecturer
School of Public Health and Clinical Sciences
University of Central Lancashire, Lancashire, UK

And

Jemma Skeat
Research Fellow
Murdoch Childrens Research Institute
Victoria, Australia

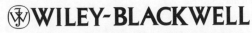WILEY-BLACKWELL

A John Wiley & Sons, Ltd., Publication

This edition first published 2010
© 2010 John Wiley & Sons Ltd

Wiley-Blackwell is an imprint of John Wiley & Sons, formed by the merger of Wiley's global
Scientific, Technical and Medical business with Blackwell Publishing.

Registered office
John Wiley & Sons Ltd, The Atrium, Southern Gate, Chichester, West Sussex, PO19 8SQ,
United Kingdom

Editorial office
John Wiley & Sons Ltd, The Atrium, Southern Gate, Chichester, West Sussex, PO19 8SQ,
United Kingdom

For details of our global editorial offices, for customer services and for information about how
to apply for permission to reuse the copyright material in this book please see our website at
www.wiley.com/wiley-blackwell.

The right of the author to be identified as the author of this work has been asserted in accordance
with the UK Copyright, Designs and Patents Act 1988.

Library of Congress Cataloging-in-Publication Data

Embedding evidence-based practice in speech and language therapy : international examples /
edited by Hazel Roddam and Jemma Skeat.
       p. ; cm.
  Includes bibliographical references and index.
  ISBN 978-0-470-74329-4 (pbk.)
1. Speech therapy.   2. Evidence-based medicine.   I. Roddam, Hazel.   II. Skeat, Jemma.
   [DNLM: 1. Speech Therapy.   2. Evidence-Based Medicine.   3. International
Cooperation.   4. Language Therapy.   WL 340.2 E53 2010]
   RC423.E56 2010
   616.85′5–dc22

                                                                          2009042695

A catalogue record for this book is available from the British Library.

Set in 10 on 12 pt Sabon by Toppan Best-set Premedia Limited
Printed and bound in Singapore by Fabulous Printers Pte Ltd

1   2010

Contents

Contributors

Sarah Beazley
Consultant Speech and Language Therapist, Cheshire and Merseyside Network for Permanent Hearing Impairment, Liverpool Primary Care Trust, UK

Leora Benjamin
Speech Pathologist, Caulfield General Medical Centre, Melbourne, Australia

Georgia D. Bertou
Speech and Language Therapist, Athens, Greece

Satty Boyes
Manager, Speech and Language Therapy Department, Salford Primary Care Trust, UK

James L. Coyle
Assistant Professor, Department of Communication Science and Disorders, University of Pittsburgh, USA

Hannah Crawford
Consultant Speech and Language Therapist, Tees, Esk and Wear Valleys NHS Trust, UK

Russell Thomas Cross
Vice President AAC Product Development, Prentke Romich Company, Wooster, OH, USA

Karen Davies
Standards Manager, Skills for Health; formerly Professional Manager for Speech and Language Therapy, Trafford Primary Care Trust, UK

Siân E. Davies
Principal Speech and Language Therapist, NHS East Lancashire, UK

Tracey C. Dean
Manager of Speech and Language Therapy Services, NHS East Lancashire, UK

Daniel De Stefanis
Speech Pathologist, Royal Melbourne Hospital, Melbourne, Australia

Angie Dobbrick
Senior Speech Pathologist, Royal Brisbane and Women's Hospital, Brisbane, Australia

Pam Enderby
*Professor of Community
Rehabilitation, School of Health and
Related Research, University of
Sheffield, UK*

Shalini Felicity Gomesz
*Speech Therapist and Teacher
Educator, Dr. Peter Bachmann
Foundation, Chilaw, Sri Lanka*

Angela Guidera
*Assistive Technology Consultant,
NovitaTech, South Australia*

Beth Higginbottom
*Speech and Language Therapist,
Victoria Hospital, Blackpool, UK*

Linda House
*Speech and Language Therapist,
Victoria Hospital, Blackpool, UK*

Tracy Kelly
*Speech Pathologist, Prince of Wales
Hospital, New South Wales, Australia*

Paula Leslie
*Associate Professor, Department of
Communication Science and
Disorders, University of Pittsburgh,
USA*

Rachel Miles Kingma
*Speech Pathologist, War Memorial
Hospital Waverley, New South Wales,
Australia*

Ruth Miller
*Speech and Language Therapist,
Manchester Primary Care Trust, UK*

Angela Morgan
*NHMRC research fellow, Murdoch
Childrens Research Institute; Senior
Speech Pathologist, Royal Children's
Hospital, Melbourne, Australia*

Patricia Oksenberg
*Speech and Language Therapist,
Levallois-Perret, France*

Catherine Olsson
*Professional Leader – Speech
Pathology, Novita Children's Services,
South Australia*

Sean Pert
*Principal Speech and Language
Therapist, Community Clinic, NHS
Heywood, Middleton and Rochdale
Community Healthcare, UK*

Parimala Raghavendra
*Manager, Research and Innovation,
Division of Research and Innovation,
Novita Children's Services, South
Australia*

Pirkko Rautakoski
*Speech and Language Therapist,
Senior Lecturer, Åbo Akademi
University, Turku, Finland*

Sheena Reilly
*Director, Speech Pathology
Department, The Royal Children's
Hospital; Professor, Paediatric Speech
Pathology, Department of Paediatrics,
The University of Melbourne; Theme
Director, Healthy Development,
Murdoch Childrens Research Institute,
Melbourne, Australia*

Rachelle Robinson
*Speech Pathologist, Prince of Wales
Hospital, New South Wales, Australia*

Hazel Roddam
*Principal Lecturer, School of Public
Health and Clinical Sciences,
University of Central Lancashire, UK*

Sheena Round
Consultant Speech and Language Therapist, Cheshire and Merseyside Network for Permanent Hearing Impairment, Liverpool Primary Care Trust, UK

Christina Samuelsson
Senior lecturer, Department of Clinical and Experimental Medicine/ Logopedics, Faculty of Health Sciences, Linköping University, Sweden

Amanda Scott
Senior Speech Pathologist, The Alfred Hospital, Melbourne, Australia

Jemma Skeat
Research Fellow, Murdoch Childrens Research Institute, Melbourne, Australia

Bea Spek
University Lecturer, Speech and Language Therapy Department, School of Health Care Studies, Hanze University Groningen, University of Applied Sciences, The Netherlands

Gina Sutcliffe
Senior Speech and Language Therapist, Speech and Language Therapy Department, Salford Primary Care Trust, UK

Gracie Tomolo
Speech Pathologist, Royal Melbourne Hospital, Melbourne, Australia

Anneli Yliherva
Speech and Language Therapist, Faculty of Humanities, Logopedics, University of Oulu, Finland

Foreword

Evidence based practice: rising to the challenge

The move to evidence-based practice (EBP) within speech and language therapy presented a challenge to clinicians, educators, researchers and our professional bodies. Some argued that EBP challenged their clinical autonomy, was too prescriptive and after all probably just another fad. Others wondered what the fuss was about because their clinical decision making was already informed by the best available scientific evidence. What's more, where evidence wasn't available, particularly for unproven techniques, they were busy systematically collecting data.

Embedding Evidence-Based Practice in Speech and Language Therapy contains numerous excellent examples of how clinicians, educators and researchers have risen to the EBP challenge. Because EBP is a life-long process of self-directed learning, formal training should begin in University courses whether at undergraduate or postgraduate level. Thus educators should be advocates for, and skilled in, EBP. Once graduates enter the workforce opportunities should exist to ensure that EBP is embedded in the way speech and language therapists think and practise.

Ensuring that the services we deliver to our clients are evidence-based means making the components of EBP 'everyone's business' as Siân Davies and Tracy Dean put it in Chapter 12. This includes participating in the evaluation of clinical practice and demonstrating that interventions used have a strong evidence base. It may also mean redesigning services to meet the needs of the community in an evidence-based way. As demonstrated by the international examples provided in this book, individuals and groups have embedded EBP into their services, practices and curricula, taking approaches that vary according to the problem being addressed and the context or environment.

Jeri Logemann writes that 'Our professions' futures depend on the effectiveness of our treatments, not on our impressions of their effectiveness'. It continues to be the responsibility of every speech pathologist whether practicing clinically, teaching or researching to narrow the knowledge–practice gap for the wellbeing of their clients and their profession.

The advent of new journals such as *Evidence Based Communication Assessment and Intervention*, have helped speech pathologists by providing succinct accessible summaries of the best evidence. In the future we need to:

1. challenge practice and teaching that is not evidence-based
2. question research that is not rigorous
3. remind those who favour experiences and impressions over science that 'the plural of anecdote is not evidence' and
4. rise to the challenge and become a collector, a collector of evidence.

It is powerful to hear about how others are participating and meeting the challenges of EBP, thereby ensuring that speech and language therapy clinical practice and teaching is grounded in the best available evidence and that our research is designed to plug some of our most critical evidence gaps.

Professor Sheena Reilly
Director, Speech Pathology Department, The Royal Children's Hospital
Professor, Paediatric Speech Pathology, Department of Paediatrics, The
    University of Melbourne
Theme Director, Healthy Development, Murdoch Childrens Research Institute,
    Melbourne, Australia

Reference

Logeman, J. What is evidence-based practice and why should we care? www.asatonline. org/resources/articles/evidencebasedpractice.htm. Accessed 24 May 2009.

Foreword

A case for professional restlessness

It is probable that most of us can identify a professional individual who we would not want to treat either ourselves or a family member. It may be a therapist that we consider out of date, a doctor who has a negative attitude, or a nurse who does not inspire confidence.

In the small hours of the morning, just before dawn, do you ever think that you may be the individual on the blacklist of a colleague? It is a salutary fact that none of us can be providing the best care to all of those in our charge all of the time. It is important that we are restless to continuously improve our patient care, student teaching, clinical management and other professional duties – but how do we do this?

The first step is to become reflective and critical reviewers of our own practice but subjectivity can lend enchantment to that perspective. Evidence-based practice can take many guises and all of the approaches described in this book can be employed by even the most busy of us to ensure that we can continue in our professional development. Even the most experienced need to be aware that experience is a two-edged sword. Experience can lead us to a confidence and familiarity with our practice which does not move on or change with new knowledge or evidence. What was best practice twelve months ago may not be so now.

Whilst randomized controlled trials (RCTs) are in the minds of many as the gold standard of evidence – which is true for some particular topics – they play a minor role in general health management and care. Most RCTs require careful selection of patients with uncomplicated diagnoses. Our clinics are mostly populated with patients who do not fit these criteria. Thus it is important to use different approaches to gather data and information to inform our practice. The broad range of methods and objectives detailed within this book should equip us to embed continual monitoring as part of our daily lives and drive us onward and upward.

Professor Pam Enderby
Professor of Community Rehabilitation
School of Health and Related Research (ScHARR)
University of Sheffield, UK

About the editors

Dr Hazel Roddam is an experienced speech and language therapist, having worked in the field of paediatric special needs and Augmentative and Alternative Communication (AAC) in the UK for over 25 years. Her PhD investigated the factors that influence the use of research in speech and language therapy. Since 2006 Hazel has worked at the University of Central Lancashire in the north-west of England, where she supervises research students across the allied health professions. Her research interests continue to focus on professional issues including promoting evidence-based practice, evaluating the impact of new roles, new ways of working and skill mix in therapy teams.

Dr Jemma Skeat is a speech pathologist and researcher. Her clinical background is in assessment, diagnosis and early intervention for children with speech and language disorders, including children with multiple and complex needs. Her PhD explored issues around the implementation and use of outcome measures by clinical speech pathologists, and her current research interests include evidence-based practice and outcome measurement in paediatric clinical services, and the use of services by families of children with speech and language needs. She currently holds an Australian National Health and Medical Research Council Postdoctoral Fellowship at the Murdoch Childrens Research Institute in Melbourne, Australia.

Acknowledgements

First and foremost, we would like to acknowledge and thank all the people who contributed chapters to this book. We were extremely fortunate to be able to find so many enthusiastic SLTs who were not only working hard to embed EBP in their clinical work, but who were also willing to share what they were doing with us and with others. We would also like to thank the people who participated in our workshop at the RCSLT Scientific Conference 2009 for their insights and fresh ideas.

There are many colleagues who have provided us with their encouragement, support, advice and expertise over the course of the development of this book – we hope that we have thanked you all individually, and that you know how important your support has been to us!

Finally, this book wouldn't have been possible without the support and patience shown to us by our families, particularly our husbands John and Wayne.

Hazel Roddam and Jemma Skeat

Section One

Understanding EBP

Purpose of this book

Hazel Roddam and Jemma Skeat

We are delighted that you have picked up this book, possibly simply out of curiosity. We hope that you will find much here to encourage you in your daily practice and possibly even to inspire you for the future. It was our intention from the outset that this should not be seen as a textbook, but rather a book that has been written by speech and language therapists (SLTs), primarily those working in clinical practice right now, in order to share their experiences with an audience of their fellow SLTs. We trust that the chapters in this book will have relevance and resonance across our professional community, whatever the clinical field, workplace setting, or geographical location. In addition we hope that this will provide a valuable resource to managers of SLT services, as well as to SLT students and those who teach them.

In fact, our aspiration for this book was articulated so clearly by two of our contributors, that we wanted to echo their words in this introduction:

> We hope that you will be able to see some similarities to your own area of expertise that will either make you feel better about your own situation or inspire you to set something similar in motion. (Sheena Round and Sarah Beazley, Chapter 13).

Background to this book

There are distinctive challenges related to evidence-based practice (EBP) for all healthcare professionals. The inspiration for this book was partly a response to these challenges. Specifically, we recognized that many SLTs still feel very unsure about what they can do as individual clinicians to embed EBP in their routine practice, and equally that managers of SLT services want to know what they can do to support their staff to more effectively embed an evidence-based approach across all aspects of their service planning and delivery. At the same time we recognize that many colleagues have been investing considerable personal effort to keep themselves as updated as they possibly can with the most recent evidence sources in their own field. It was this that first inspired us to seek a way to share all these insights with a wider audience.

It was a considerable challenge to select only a relatively few examples for inclusion in this book. We know that there are many other positive and innovative approaches – and we hope that this publication will prompt more active dissemination of many more ideas on this topic via a range of channels. As you read the following contributions, we would ask you to recognize the spirit in which these chapters have been offered. It was our aspiration that these contributed chapters should represent a broad geographical spread, as well as a wide range of work settings; from services that are situated within large organizations, such as hospitals, to SLTs working together in agencies, to sole independent practitioners. It is the universal interest of any healthcare staff to focus on their own preferred clinical topics and SLTs excel in networking with fellow clinicians in their own clinical specialism. In our invited chapters we have also endeavoured to achieve a spread across this dimension, from paediatrics to adult, and across speech, language, voice, fluency, dysphagia, alternative and augmentative communication (AAC) and other clinical areas.

Naturally it has not been possible to be exhaustive in representing all contexts, clinical areas and geographic locations, but we hope that you will find it exciting to discover how much we all share the same perspectives and concerns wherever we are, and whatever the setting in which we are working.

In preparing for this book we had to make a decision regarding the choice of professional title that we judged would be most familiar and inclusive to an international audience. We are well aware that Speech–Language Pathologist is the preferred term in the US, Canada and in Asia; Speech Pathologist in Australia; and Speech and Language Therapist in the UK, South Africa and New Zealand. Across the countries of mainland Europe there are of course local titles to describe the job role, many derived from *Orthophoniste–Logopede*. In many cases these titles have been established through a process of professional regulation. The debates regarding the influence of the title on our professional identity as well as on public perceptions cannot be underestimated, and we have been mindful of that in our deliberations. Since our book contains contributions from many corners of the world, we felt that that our primary consideration should simply be to go for consistency across the book and to avoid the need for cumbersome duplication. For the purpose of sharing the messages in this book, we trust that our choice of Speech and Language Therapist (SLT) will be acceptable across the whole professional community.

How this book is organized

We have attempted to draw together contributions that address specific challenges in relation to embedding EBP in the profession. The chapters are organized to address each of these broad challenges, which are:

- Understanding why EBP is important to SLTs and what some of the major barriers are (Section One)
- Developing skills and knowledge for EBP (Section Two)
- Creating a supportive context for EBP (Section Three)

- Making the evidence work for us (Section Four)
- Understanding how evidence can be applied to meet clinical challenges (Section Five)
- Future directions for EBP (Section Six)

The aim of this introduction is to provide you with a brief overview of these sections, and each of the chapters within.

Challenge one: Understanding EBP and the barriers to embedding EBP

We felt that it was imperative to begin this book with a clear definition of EBP, plus some consideration of the factors that are known to support or to constrain EBP. Chapter 2 provides a definition of EBP, making a clear distinction between research activity, research use and an evidence-based approach to practice. Chapter 3 provides an overview of the growing research around factors that have been identified to act as barriers and facilitators for embedding EBP across healthcare groups, and particularly for the allied health professions (AHP).

Challenge two: Addressing specific skills gaps and meeting training needs

Many SLTs still identify that they have training needs related to EBP. These particularly relate to finding and appraising published research evidence, but also include skills in implementing evidence-based changes in their day-to-day work – and then in subsequently measuring the effectiveness of those changes in practice. In this section we showcase four approaches to developing skills and knowledge in EBP with two chapters focussing on formal approaches via undergraduate and postgraduate education, and two chapters describing initiatives to facilitate the ongoing development of staff skills in the clinical setting.

Chapter 4 is about an undergraduate SLT course at Hanze University in the Netherlands, which uses a highly structured developmental approach to EBP to match the learning needs of students preparing to embark on their career in SLT.

Chapter 5 focuses on a how postgraduate training in Pittsburg, USA introduces a rigorous approach to EBP for SLTs who are already experienced in clinical practice.

Chapter 6 introduces a Clinical Effectiveness Group, designed to be 'more than a journal club' for a UK hospital-based SLT service, with the purpose of building EBP skills and confidence in staff.

Chapter 7 demonstrates the value of mentorship in EBP, through a system of clinical supervision. This initiative is located in the UK, in a specialist dysphagia service for adults with learning difficulty.

Chapter 8 is our chance to comment on these initiatives, referring readers to a number of excellent sources that support the development of EBP skills and knowledge.

Challenge three: Working in a supportive context

The next challenge that faces us all is the influence of the context in which we work. The chapters in this section reflect a range of factors that have been identified as contributing to a workplace or organizational culture, which may either facilitate or constrain progress in embedding an EBP approach by clinicians. In this section there are a wide range of approaches which have been implemented within SLT services to support and to promote evidence-based service planning and service delivery.

Chapter 9 describes the essential role of clinical leadership, written by an experienced manager of a large SLT service. It presents her approach to developing a culture of learning, and illustrates how she engages the clinicians in undertaking evidence-based service planning.

Chapter 10 provides an example of how evidence-based service redesign (in this case, prompted by a recognition of the pressures on SLTs to manage ever-growing caseloads) can support clinical staff to take a closer look at their own practice, and to realign what they do with the evidence.

Chapter 11 relates a model of clinical research support that has been running in South Australia for over ten years. As part of this, joint clinician–research positions have been created to facilitate undertaking of research projects in a community-based clinical setting.

Chapter 12 suggests a way to celebrate EBP, promoting the development of a positive culture. These authors describe their Professional Development Forum, which has been used promote and celebrate EBP initiatives across all the clinical teams within their service.

Chapter 13 is a further contribution from UK that presents the development of a highly specialist region-wide service for children with a profound hearing impairment. The authors discuss the way that evidence was used to shape the design of the new service, and how the new service has supported clinicians to embed EBP.

Chapter 14 includes a brief overview of recent work using a benchmarking methodology, to measure contextual factors that are known to support EBP.

Challenge four: Making the evidence work for us

There are many ways that clinicians and managers alike can support the practical accessibility of the evidence. Access to the evidence is not just about how many online journals your institution subscribes to. Practical evidence-based resources such as evidence-based guidelines, policies, assessment tools and summaries of the 'clinical bottom line' of papers are essential for busy practitioners. In this section we include some examples of how SLTs have tackled the development of these resources. Additionally, we consider the tools that exist to support us to access client views, a key part of the evidence that we need to consider.

Chapter 15 focuses on incorporating the views of service users, and describes ways that this can be done through various existing SLT-specific tools. This chapter contribution challenges us to consider what we are currently doing to make our services 'client focused'.

Chapter 16 describes the development of an evidence-based assessment tool. This tool is intended to specifically meet the needs of SLTs working with clients who use AAC, and who need a tool to enable reflection on client progress.

Chapter 17 demonstrates the development and implementation of an evidence-based policy which is used to ensure that clinical staff adhere to the evidence for safe and effective dysphagia assessment in a hospital setting.

Chapter 18 showcases an initiative that supports SLT clinicians from different physical locations, clinical settings and backgrounds to share the task of critical appraisal for the development of practical, evidence-based summaries of single papers and topics.

Chapter 19 provides a discussion of other ways that we can 'equip' ourselves for EBP by bringing together the research evidence in a form that is easy to understand and relevant to the ins and outs of our clinical situation.

Challenge five: Understanding how the evidence can be applied to meet clinical challenges

For many of us, it is not easy to access a clear appreciation of how our professional colleagues are working around the world. While the previous sections have focused on individual and organizational strategies for embedding EBP, we also wanted this book to provide some clear clinical examples of what EBP looks like in real life: times when clinicians have faced a particular clinical question, and have accessed and implemented the evidence in their own clinical situation.

Section Five includes a breadth of scenarios that reflect many clinical fields of SLT practice. Whilst it was never going to be possible for this to be exhaustive, we feel that this compilation reflects many areas of clinical practice. Nevertheless we would like these examples to be considered not just in light of their clinical field, but also in terms of the challenges that are highlighted and the strategies that these clinicians used when approaching and implementing the evidence to meet their clinical needs. These challenges and strategies are relevant to more than just a single clinical area.

We are also delighted that these contributions represent a significantly wide geographical range, particularly including a number of countries across mainland Europe, as well as from Asia and Australia. This generates a particularly valuable opportunity to reflect on the broader influences on the delivery of our SLT services. For this reason we asked all our contributors to open their chapters by setting the scene.

Challenge six: Looking ahead to the future

This final section of the book comprises a slightly wider perspective on the issue of embedding EBP in SLT practice. As one part of this process we undertook a small-scale workshop activity at an international conference to elicit additional comments from members of the profession.

Chapter 32 describes the workshop event and summarizes the themes that were generated. These themes and the illustrative examples from participants are presented to complement the challenges we have already identified in the preceding sections. We also report on an additional focus that comprised proposals that were made for the professional associations to take an increasingly strategic role in promoting EBP for their members.

Chapter 33 focuses on the link between reflective practice and EBP, as this theme was particularly highlighted by the workshop participants. Ways of supporting 'reflection' in everyday clinical practice, as suggested by participants, were developing routines for accessing and reading new literature, and using clinical audit and outcome measures to evaluate the processes and outcomes of clinical practice. We discuss these strategies and provide some practical suggestions.

Chapter 34 brings this book to a close with our thoughts on what should be the next priorities for our profession. In particular we focus on the potential for sharing good practice initiatives for service-user engagement, plus considering how we can engage with our colleagues from other disciplines, in recognition of the multidisciplinary nature of much of our work.

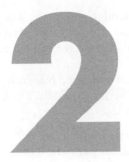

What does EBP mean to speech and language therapists?

Hazel Roddam and Jemma Skeat

Evidence-based practice (EBP) has been the growing mantra across healthcare services since early in the 1990s. Most of us feel that we have a perception of what this means, but how confidently can we demonstrate that this has become a fundamental element of our professional identity? Is EBP integral to our daily routine, and not simply a luxury to be contemplated when we have the time and the energy at the end of our busy clinics? We feel that it is essential to start this book with some clearly articulated definitions of what EBP is agreed to be – and what it is not. We will also present a well-established stage model for implementing an EBP approach in clinical practice. As you read the contributed chapters in each section of this book, you will be able to see how these real-life examples relate to the definitions presented here. We appreciate that for some readers the issues covered in this chapter will be more familiar than for others. There is limited space in this chapter for exhaustive examination of all the relevant issues, but we hope that our comments will provide a structured framework for reflecting on all the subsequent messages in this book.

Defining EBP

We have each noted when talking to colleagues that there still exists a degree of uncertainty and ambiguity surrounding the distinction between being an evidence-based practitioner and being research-active. Throughout this book we will show how much our profession depends upon high quality research that has direct applications to our clinical practice. We need experienced clinicians to collaborate closely with researchers to contribute to our collective research base, and some of those will go on to become confident and accomplished independent researchers. But the purpose of this book is not to encourage speech and language therapists (SLTs) to consider whether that will be their path: our aim to is emphasize that it is essential for us to keep ourselves updated with the research in our own field and to ensure that we use it to underpin our clinical decision-making. We would echo the assertion made in Culyer's working party recommendations to the UK Department of Health on this issue: that it is not expected that all healthcare staff should be research active, but it is deemed that they should be active users of research (Culyer, 1994).

Now that we have made a distinction between doing research and using research, we want to move onto clarifying what we mean by EBP. The most widely cited definition of EBP is that published by Sackett *et al.* (1996, p. 2):

> 'evidence based medicine is the conscientious, judicious and explicit use of current best evidence in making the decisions about individual patients. The practice of evidence based medicine means integrating individual clinical expertise with the best available evidence from systematic research'.

Subsequent authors have broadened the application of this definition of evidence-based medicine to other healthcare professionals (Bury and Mead, 1998), as well as to other healthcare aspects, including commissioning and purchasing, policy management and patient choice (Muir-Gray, 2001; Stewart, 2002). Sackett emphasized that the use of research evidence was intended to support expert clinical judgement (Sackett *et al.*, 1996), to counter the criticisms that EBP was perceived to be overly prescriptive and threatened professional and clinical autonomy (Bury and Mead, 1998; Closs and Cheater, 1999).

We would like to highlight the difference between EBP and research utilization (RU). RU has been defined as 'the clinical application of some portion of research in a way similar to that was used in the original study' (Polit and Hungler, 1999). In contrast, EBP is the more extensive process of incorporating the evaluation of a range of evidence sources to explicitly inform daily clinical practice (Taylor, 2000). For this reason it is important that the terms RU and EBP are used judiciously and are not perceived to be interchangeable. We share the concerns of Papps (2003) that until the terminology is transparent across the profession, EBP will not be embraced whole-heartedly. If we want to convince our colleagues to become more 'evidence-based', then we have to be able to communicate clearly about what we should all be aiming for, and be able to have a way of benchmarking our progress towards that: otherwise, how will we know when we are 'there'?

What are the drivers for EBP?

EBP grew from the evidence-based medicine (EBM) movement in the 1970s and 1980s. During this time the authority of health care professionals to define good patient care had weakened, as studies showed that even 'experts' in health care did not agree on how health care should be practised (Enzmann, 1997), and the public's knowledge of health care increased (Wessen, 1999). Third parties, such as governments and health care insurance providers, were beginning to demand factual evidence, rather than clinical wisdom, as the basis on which to make decisions about effective care (Starfield, 1985; Hansen, Mior and Mootz, 2000). Claims regarding both competence and effectiveness required credible data (Hansen *et al.*, 2000). EBM is now a 'fundamental element in Western-style clinical medicine' (Reilly, Douglas and Oates, 2004, p. 4). EBM contrasts with traditional approaches across clinical practice that had previously been largely based on historical antecedents and unsubstantiated opinions, perpetuated through apprenticeship-style professional training: 'most of what we do, we do because we do it' (Baker, 1998, p. 35). It has also been contrasted with decision making by anecdote, by press-cutting or by expert opinion (Greenhalgh, 1997); all of which can be seen now to comprise significant weaknesses in terms of assuring patient safety, as well as standardized quality of care.

The growth of EBM in clinical medicine has been mirrored within the allied health profession (AHP) groups where there has also been an increasing emphasis that the basis of clinical decision-making needs to focus explicitly more on high quality evidence than on clinical experience and intuition (Enderby and Emerson, 1995; Bury and Mead, 1998; Reilly et al., 2004). SLTs, like other healthcare professionals are experiencing pressures to demonstrate that they are providing effective and efficient services, and showing a strong commitment to EBP is integral to this. Professional associations have actively promoted the use of EBP over the past decade and this is linked both with regulatory requirements for continuing professional development (CPD) and with clinical effectiveness (Yorkston et al., 2001). Many of the SLT associations world-wide now have professional standards that reference EBP: for example in the UK context, the Royal College of Speech and Language Therapists stated the aspiration that EBP should become 'embedded in speech and language therapy at all levels' (RCSLT, 2003, p. 2). It was further specified that each SLT service should have 'a strategic and systematic approach within each clinical team to establish an evidence-based resource as the basis for provision of clinical care, organization of services and service development' (RCSLT, 2006, p. 116).

What constitutes the 'evidence' and where should we look for it?

There have been extensive debates over what constitutes evidence (Bury and Mead, 1998). EBP is intended to comprise three distinctive strands: the research evidence base, our clinical expertise, plus a consideration of the service user's unique circumstances or preferences regarding their care (Sackett et al., 1996). Several authors have suggested a fourth category: relevant information from the local context (Schlosser, 2003; Rycroft-Malone et al., 2004). Therefore, the definition of 'evidence' is much broader than just research data. It also encompasses patient assessment and outcomes data, the views and preferences of our service users, information about the complexity of the context, and our own clinical opinions (Sackett et al., 1996; DH, 1997; McCormack et al., 2002; Schlosser, 2003). In fact, it may be maintained that there could be little justification for excluding any type of information in decision making in clinical care, provided that an appraisal has been made of its relevance and validity.

We also need to remember that research evidence varies, and while there has been a traditional focus on prioritizing the value of experimental research evidence, we cannot afford to ignore all sources of research evidence other than randomized controlled trials. For example, Enderby and Emerson (1995) highlighted that we need to undertake mixed-method studies where the advantages of both qualitative and quantitative approaches can be combined.

Just as the 'evidence' that we use needs to be broad, so, too, should our searches for the evidence. On the other hand, given the time pressures that are an inevitable part of our work, it is essential that SLTs are able to access this evidence as effectively and efficiently as possible. The use of pre-appraised evidence sources, such as systematic reviews – including those published by the Cochrane Collaboration – are essential to support SLTs to use evidence in practice. Well-conducted systematic reviews present a synthesis of studies that have all been appraised for the quality of design and rigour of conduct and hence can provide a sound basis to support clinicians. There are references in Chapter 8 to sources of guidance on how to appraise the quality of a systematic review. Several of our chapter authors also discuss issues relevant to accessing the evidence, and Section Four of the book focuses on building resources and methods that 'make the evidence work for us', for example, by the development and use of secondary sources of evidence, such as evidence-based clinical guidelines and policies.

We cannot end this section without a note about issues related to the current evidence base for SLT. There continues to be some variability in both the volume and quality of research evidence across the clinical specialisms (Enderby and Emerson, 1995; Reilly et al., 2004) and this is a concern that has been frequently reported by therapists (Metcalfe et al., 2001). On the other hand, having included examples from authors around the world in this book has reminded us that there are substantial evidence bases in other languages that have not all been translated into English. Here is yet another challenge to us all to be more conscious of recognizing that there may be other very relevant evidence bases that we are not currently accessing (Reynolds, 2009).

It will be inevitable that we will all face clinical challenges where there is an apparent dearth in the research literature. But that is by no means a reason to feel reluctant to engage in EBP. As the evidence base grows there will increasingly be relevant sources. However, in the meanwhile we hope that SLTs will be encouraged to take what does exist and use it to inform their treatment, alongside patient opinions and their own clinical expertise. It was for this reason that Roddam (2004) suggested that we should consider describing our case management choices as being 'evidence-informed' rather than 'evidence-based'.

We cannot emphasize enough the importance of considering EBP as more than just 'using research'. Simply referencing research for treatment efficacy does not in itself constitute EBP without due consideration of the other strands. In fact, Schlosser and Sigafoos (2008) argued that it is only in applying assessment or treatment approaches to the care of a particular patient, and taking into account our own clinical knowledge and patient preferences, that these approaches can be called 'evidence-based'. They suggest that we should think about assessment or treatment modes that have proven efficacy through rigorous research as 'empirically-supported' or 'empirically-validated'.

Despite the above considerations about terminology, we have chosen to use the term 'evidence-based practice' throughout the book as this is currently more familiar to SLTs than 'evidence-informed practice'. However, we think that there is value in the profession considering the message that it communicates about the approaches that we use and how these are applied in our practice, through terms such as EBP, 'evidence informed' and 'empirically supported treatment'.

Practising EBP: The EBP stage model

The most widely used model for EBP is that published by Sackett *et al.* (1997). His model was presented as a five-stage cycle, to lead clinicians through the entire process. These steps direct the clinician to:

- formulate a clinical question, either about an individual patient or a client group
- search for relevant high quality evidence
- critically appraise the evidence for rigour of design and conduct
- implement changes in clinical practice if appropriate
- evaluate practice and disseminate the findings.

There is a need to accept that this will necessarily be an iterative, cyclical undertaking, for two reasons. First, there is the need to stay current with the generation of new knowledge; which for some clinical areas may prove to be more rapidly changing than others. Second, we need to guard against complacency in our own practice: having adopted new practices based on relevant research evidence, we need to ensure that we maintain those standards and do not revert to former ways of working.

There have been many subsequent publications that have incorporated well-written guides to support clinicians to undertake this process and this is discussed further in Chapter 8.

Embedding EBP – what are the challenges?

The expectation that there will be an inevitable cascade effect of research knowledge into clinical practice has been shown to be excessively simplistic and essentially unpredictable (Dopson *et al.*, 2002). The inherent challenges of EBP for all healthcare professionals comprise the need for a quality research evidence base, plus the skills and organizational support to utilize those research findings. EBP presents a challenge to us all, and we need to consider how best to meet this challenge by ensuring that we are appropriately skilled and equipped, with cultures and contexts that embrace EBP. We present a discussion about the barriers to embedding EBP – and what we might be able to do to overcome them – in the next chapter.

References

Baker, M. (1998) Taking the strategy forward. In M. Baker and S. Kirk (Eds.), *Research and Development for the NHS: Evidence, Evaluation and Effectiveness* (2nd edn). Oxford: Radcliffe Medical Press.

Bury, T. and Mead, J. (1998) *Evidence-based Healthcare: A Practical Guide for Therapists.* Oxford: Butterworth-Heinemann.

Closs, S.J. and Cheater, F.M. (1999) Evidence for nursing practice: a clarification of the issues. *Journal of Advanced Nursing*, **30** (1), 10–17.

Culyer, A.J. (1994) *Supporting research and development in the NHS: a report to the Minister for Health by a research and Development Task Force chaired by Professor Anthony Culyer.* London: HMSO.

Department of Health (1997) *The New NHS: Modern, Dependable.* London: HMSO.

Dopson, S., FitzGerald, L., Ferlie, E., Gabbay, J. and Locock, L. (2002) No magic targets! Changing clinical practice to become more evidence-based. *Health Care Management Review*, **27** (3), 35–47.

Enderby, P. and Emerson, J. (1995) *Does Speech and Language Therapy Work? A Review of the Literature.* London: Whurr.

Enzmann, D.R. (1997) *Surviving in Health Care.* St Louis, MO: Mosby.

Greenhalgh, T. (1997) *How to Read a Paper: The Basics of Evidence-Based Medicine.* London: BMJ.

Hansen, D.T., Mior, S. and Mootz, R.D. (2000) Why outcomes? Why now? In S.G. Yeomans (ed.), *The clinical application of outcomes assessment* (pp. 3–14). Stamford, CT: Appleton and Lange.

McCormack, B., Kitson, A., Harvey, G., Rycroft-Malone, J., Titchen, A. and Seers, K. (2002) Getting evidence into practice: the meaning of 'context'. *Journal of Advanced Nursing* **38** (1), 94–104.

Metcalfe, C., Lewin, R., Wisher, S., Perry, S., Bannigan, K. and Moffett, J.K. (2001) Barriers to implementing the evidence-base in four NHS therapies: Dieticians, occupational therapists, physiotherapists, speech and language therapists. *Physiotherapy*, **87** (8), 433–441.

Muir-Gray, J.A. (2001) *Evidence-Based Healthcare: How to Make Health Policy and Management Decisions* (2nd edn). London: Churchill Livingstone.

Papps, E. (2003) *Conversations in a sandpit: the language of evidence-based practice.* Paper presented at the Evidence in Practice Conference, Bristol, UK.

Polit, D. and Hungler, B.P. (1999) *Nursing Research: Principles and Methods.* New York: Lippincott.

Reilly, S., Douglas, J. and Oates, J. (2004) *Evidence Based Practice in Speech Pathology.* London: Whurr.

Reynolds, J. (2009) Plus ca change, or vive la difference? *RCSLT Bulletin*, March, 20.

Roddam, H. (2004) The efficacy of augmentative and alternative communication: Towards evidence-based practice (Editorial). *Communication Matters*, **18** (2), 23–24.

Royal College of Speech and Language Therapists (2003) *Research and Development Strategy (final draft).* London: RCSLT.

Royal College of Speech and Language Therapists (2006) *Communicating Quality 3.* London: RCSLT.

Rycroft-Malone, J., Seers, K., Titchen, A., Harvey, G., Kitson, A. and McCormack, B. (2004) What counts as evidence in evidence-based practice? *Journal of Advanced Nursing*, **47** (1), 81–90.

Sackett, D.L., Rosenberg, W.M.C., Gray, J.A.M., Haynes, R.B. and Richardson, W.S. (1996) Evidence-based medicine: What it is and what it isn't. *British Medical Journal*, **312**, 71–72.

Sackett, D.L., Richardson, W.S., Rosenberg, W. and Haynes, R.B. (1997) *Evidence-Based Medicine: How to Practice and Teach EBM.* London: Churchill Livingstone.

Schlosser, R. (2003) *The Efficacy of Augmentative and Alternative Communication: Toward Evidence-Based Practice*. San Diego: Academic Press.

Schlosser, R.W. and Sigafoos, J. (2008) Identifying 'evidence-based practice' versus 'empirically supported treatment' (Editorial). *Evidence-Based Communication Assessment and Intervention*, **2**, 2, 61–62.

Starfield, B. (1985) *The Effectiveness of Medical Care: Validating Clinical Wisdom*. Baltimore: Johns Hopkins.

Stewart, R. (2002) *Evidence-based Management: A Practical Guide for Health Professionals*. Abingdon: Radcliffe Medical Press.

Taylor, M. (2000) *Evidence-based Practice for Occupational Therapists*. Oxford: Blackwell Science.

Wessen, A.F. (1999) The comparitive study of health care reform. In F.D. Powell and A.F. Wessen (eds), *Health Care Systems in Transition: An International Perspective*. Thousand Oaks, CA: Sage, pp. 3–24.

Yorkston, K.M., Spencer, K., Duffy, J., *et al*. (2001) Evidence-based medicine and practice guidelines: Application to the field of speech-language pathology. *Journal of Medical Speech-Language Pathology*, **9**, 243–256.

What are the barriers to EBP in speech and language therapy?

Jemma Skeat and Hazel Roddam

The previous chapter has clarified a definition of evidence-based practice (EBP), and has discussed why this is so important for speech and language therapists (SLTs) around the world. The arguments for taking an evidence-based approach to our care of clients with communication and swallowing needs are compelling, but there is a large and ever-growing body of research that suggests that implementing an evidence-based approach to practice is difficult for health care professionals across many fields. EBP requires change to habits, routines, and sometimes personal and philosophical preferences and ideals. The purpose of this chapter is to present an overview of this body of relevant work, to help readers to consider some of the known barriers to EBP plus the existing evidence for overcoming these barriers. Understanding barriers in your own setting may help you when considering EBP initiatives, perhaps inspired by some of the examples provided by the clinicians who have contributed to this book.

Is there really a research–practice gap?

The transfer of research knowledge into practice has been emphasized as being essential to improve patient care and service delivery (Department of Health, 1995), but it has been acknowledged that there is a gap between research evidence and clinical practice across all healthcare organizations (Rosenberg and Donald, 1995). Research into speech and language therapy uptake of EBP has shown that not all SLTs are regularly accessing research findings and the translation of research recommendations into clinical practice is highly variable, with as few as 18% or as many as 80% of SLTs reporting that they frequently use research evidence to inform patient care (Vallino-Napoli and Reilly, 2004; Zipoli and Kennedy, 2005), depending on which study you access. For those who are not, or who are only infrequently using the evidence to inform practice, what might the barriers be?

Firstly, it may be a question of attitudes or perceptions about EBP. There are a number of models used frequently in the psychological and social sciences that suggest that people's attitudes influence their behaviour (Ajzen, 1991, 2002), and therefore, understanding and addressing these attitudes is important.

Secondly, we may feel that we lack the necessary skills or knowledge needed in order to find the right evidence, to understand the content, and to critically appraise and apply the evidence to practice.

Thirdly, it may be that we don't feel that we have time to read, process and consider the implications for this new evidence, and to make practice changes when needed.

Fourthly, accessing the evidence may be a problem. This is not just a question of having access to the right journals: our client's views are also part of EBP and accessing these views can present a challenge, particularly when clients have communication difficulties. The evidence itself can present a challenge, for example, in the way that it is reported, often with complex statistics and sometimes with little emphasis on the clinical bottom line. Sometimes the information that we need to answer a clinical question just doesn't exist.

Finally, if the evidence suggests a change to practice is needed, there may be specific barriers that exist that make this difficult to achieve, such as a lack of support from management.

For all of the above barriers, organizational and cultural factors can be very influential. For example, a supportive context for EBP may influence SLTs to have positive attitudes, and such a context may be more likely to provide resources that are necessary to access the evidence, or training to support the development of appropriate skills. The barriers above are also interlinked, for example, knowledge and skills can influence attitudes and can reduce the time needed to access and use the evidence. All of these barriers are considered below, as well as some suggestions around overcoming them.

Barriers to EBP

Perceptions of EBP

Several recent surveys across allied health profession (AHP) groups have indicated generally positive perceptions of the principles of EBP (including Upton, 1999; Metcalfe et al., 2001; Pennington, 2001; Vallino-Napoli and Reilly, 2004; Zipoli and Kennedy, 2005). In contrast, studies that use more in-depth evaluation of AHP perceptions about EBP, for example using qualitative interviews, have reported that staff expressed considerable uncertainties and reservations about how they were expected to be implementing these principles (Roddam, 2003; Tse et al., 2004). There is even evidence that some of us feel a sense of guilt about prioritizing time for EBP activities (such as reading and appraising research literature) over direct contact time with clients (Lankshear, 2002; Roddam, 2003; Wilks and Boniface, 2004).

Research has shown that people's attitudes are a good predictor of their intentions to implement evidence in practice (Walker et al., 2004; Bonetti et al., 2005). In fact, 'changes in attitudes are likely to be important in bringing about sustained changes in behaviour [of health care professionals], which may ultimately benefit care of patients' (Coomarasamy and Khan, 2004).

There has recently been a growing awareness that clinicians' perceptions of EBP are underpinned by their personal values and beliefs and that these are also related to their professional role and to their perceptions of what it means to involve patients in decision making (Fish and Coles, 1998; van der Gaag and Mowles, 2005). Specific experiences and exposure at critical times in training and professional development may also play an important role. Zipoli and Kennedy (2005) reported that exposure to research during undergraduate training, and the practical demonstration of the use of research in the workplace in the early years of clinical practice strongly impacted on SLTs' personal attitudes towards EBP. The place in which we work may be important, as these researchers also found distinct differences of perceptions were reported by SLTs who worked in the community compared to those in the hospital-based teams. This finding resonates with Kennedy's (2002) distinction between the approaches to communication disorders of these two groups, where there continues to be a degree of conflict between a social model and a medical model of professional culture.

Psychological theories also highlight the importance of our underlying beliefs in influencing attitudes (Ajzen, 1991, 2002). For example, if we believe that accessing, reading and applying the evidence to our practice will lead to tangible and important benefits for patients, then our attitudes to EBP are likely to be positive. Similarly, if we believe that EBP is something scary, difficult and unlikely to lead to important changes, then our attitudes are likely to be negative. Our beliefs are influenced by our experiences and the experiences of others, which is why it is important for SLTs to demonstrate and share with one another the positive benefits of using evidence-based approaches, including tangible outcomes data where relevant. We also suggest that a primary target in any EBP-promoting strategy should be to ensure that all SLTs have an unambiguous understanding of EBP principles and processes, plus a clear perception of how they are expected to apply this to their own clinical practice. It is important that SLTs understand the principle that EBP is not intended to undermine their clinical judgement, experience and expertise, but to support it (Sackett et al., 1996).

Skills for EBP

There are numerous studies across AHP groups indicating that staff perceived they lacked key skills for EBP, including a significant lack of confidence in independent reading and critical appraisal of research reports (Taylor, 2000; Metcalfe et al., 2001; Upton and Upton, 2006). Some of the issues around negative personal attitudes towards EBP may well be founded in low confidence in these skills, which include awareness of research designs, searching of electronic databases, critical appraisal of research papers, and implementing and measuring clinical change. SLTs need to be proficient in judging the evidence with confidence, to determine whether it is valid, reliable and relevant to their own clinical circumstances. It is also essential that SLTs understand that they need to guard against drawing the wrong conclusions from published studies. We should only consider changing our clinical practice when we are fully satisfied that the research evidence is appropriate to our own local clinical circumstances, and when we have considered it alongside our own clinical knowledge and the preferences of patients.

Identifying and addressing these skills gaps needs to be an essential component of a systematic approach to supporting EBP (Stetler, 2003). Following initial training in EBP skills, maintenance of therapists' confidence appears to be the next challenge, with indications that regular practice in critical appraisal of research articles is essential to achieving this (Bannigan and Hooper, 2002). There are a number of ways that this can be achieved, including journal clubs, mentoring and clinical supervision, participating in interest groups and other networks where critical appraisal is undertaken, and the use of formal continuing education programmes. Making use of external resources, for example, via links to local universities, can provide access to expertise and skills which can be fruitful in supporting EBP locally. Collaborative efforts, whereby clinical SLTs raise and prioritize the salient clinical questions to steer the direction of much needed applied clinical research could be one benefit of this approach, which would not only expose clinicians to research skills but add to the evidence base. Some of these approaches are illustrated by contributors in this book.

Time for EBP

Unsurprisingly, time for reading research and time for implementing practice changes were major barriers, reported without exception in all of the empirical studies with AHPs (Closs and Lewin, 1998; Pollock *et al.*, 2000; Pennington, 2001, Metcalfe *et al.*, 2001; Vallino-Napoli and Reilly, 2004; Zipoli and Kennedy, 2005), as well as in studies evaluating EBP in other professions such as nursing (Walsh, 1997; Dunn *et al.*, 1998; Kajermo *et al.*, 1998; Law and Baum, 1998; McCleary and Brown, 2003; Veeramah, 2004). Concerns about time may be well-founded, as Brackenbury and colleagues (2008) demonstrated that searching for and evaluating the evidence for a hypothetical speech and language therapy clinical case took between three and seven hours to complete.

Prioritizing the time that we have available to us is important, as it is unlikely that we are all going to be able to access extra hours in the day. There are numerous strategies that support clinicians to be more efficient and effective in EBP activities, such as accessing the evidence – for example, using journal alerts to help us identify new relevant research. There are indications of clear benefits where we can undertake appraisal of research literature with colleagues; most particularly when the selection of topics is determined by clinical priorities, thus sustaining motivation to attend and participate. This group appraisal activity is similar to some models of a journal club, but the emphasis needs to be soundly based on real and current clinical questions as prioritized by the participants; as was specifically recommended by Coomarasamy and Khan (2004) for the medical profession, as well as by Bannigan and Hooper (2002) for AHPs. Additionally, the evidence may support us to reconsider and redevelop our services so that we work more efficiently, are less over overwhelmed by our clinical caseloads and more likely to find time for EBP. Again, we are happy to say that a number of examples in this book illustrate these time-saving strategies.

Access to research evidence

Access to research information was one of the four main factors specified by Funk and colleagues (1991) in their seminal work on identifying barriers to research use for nurses. SLTs have specified several resource issues as presenting serious constraints to their use of research evidence (Metcalfe *et al.*, 2001; Zipoli and Kennedy, 2005; Upton and Upton, 2006). They cited access to IT facilities, as well as access to copies of full research papers, rather than only abstracts found via electronic databases. This clearly constitutes a substantially greater difficulty for SLT staff working in some settings than in others. In general, staff working on hospital sites may be able to benefit more from access to local medical library services, which are less available to staff in community-based services. On the other hand, access may be a decreasing barrier, due to the widespread use of the internet across health care organizations. Gosling and Westbrook (2004) reported on AHPs' use of online evidence in New South Wales, finding that 76% of their 790 respondents had used online evidence.

Accessing the evidence is not just about being able to locate journal articles. There a number of issues around the research evidence itself, which can present significant barriers to EBP. One cannot access evidence that doesn't exist, and there are notable gaps in the evidence base for some areas of SLT practice (Gillam and Gillam, 2006). The evidence that does exist is of variable quality and strength and the way that research findings are presented can be difficult to understand and relate to clinical practice (Metcalfe *et al.*, 2001). In fact, a number of sources have indicated a prevalent perception across SLTs that published research often does not sufficiently focus on clinically relevant topics, nor sufficiently emphasize the clinical applications of research findings (Ingram, 1998; Pennington, 2001; Enderby, 2004). SLTs also stated that they found research reports difficult to read and to evaluate (Closs and Lewin, 1998; Upton, 1999; Pennington, 2001).

In all circumstances, it is essential that issues related to accessing research literature are acknowledged and addressed, otherwise EBP cannot become embedded as a fundamental component of SLT culture.

Supportive context and culture

As described in the previous chapter, implementing EBP represents the full cycle of identifying the need for a service change, adopting that change, and then evaluating the impact of that change. The context in which SLTs work is an essential part of this cycle. A number of studies have indicated the influence of context or culture on research use in practice (Taylor, 2000; Pennington *et al.*, 2005). These findings support the influence of the leadership role in promoting a positive culture, as described first by Rogers (1995) and Handy (1999). These factors have been further reinforced for healthcare services by the conceptual frameworks developed by Kitson *et al.* (1998) and by Stetler (2003). Empirical work (Roddam, 2003) has also specifically highlighted the influence of SLT service managers in leading a positive research culture, by the way in which they authorize and value EBP activities and related initiatives. This further serves to reinforce the importance of a work context where there is explicit strategic use of research evidence (Stetler, 2003). However, one of the major challenges continues to be the validation of measures to evaluate the research climate, or culture, of healthcare departments and teams (Baker, 1998). These issues are discussed further in Chapter 14.

Some research has indicated that there are potential benefits to the culture of a department or group generated by working alongside colleagues who are research-active, possibly as they are perceived to be 'educationally influential' (Oxman *et al.*, 1995). Such individuals may also prove to be appropriate candidates to act as EBP 'champions' – providing EBP leadership in clinical practice. However, it has been recognized that research-active staff may also potentially generate a negative influence (Dopson *et al.*, 2002; Roddam, 2003), causing other staff to feel even more daunted by their perceptions of the research agenda. It seems that service managers need to ensure positive support for staff who are, or who wish to become research-active and to remain alert to these issues.

Context and culture can promote or impede all aspects of EBP. In fact, while most of the research into barriers for EBP has so far focused on individual aspects, there is a growing sense that there needs to be more emphasis on the organizational level (MacGuire, 2006). A number of studies appear to indicate that the organization may be more influential in determining whether or not EBP is embedded (Dopson *et al.*, 2002). It is easy to see why this is the case. Even when considering individual factors, such as knowledge or skills, the organization in which they work plays a key role in whether or not SLTs can access things like training, mentoring, and so on. Context and culture are also crucial influences on whether or not SLTs are able to make changes to their clinical work on the basis of the evidence.

Overcoming the research–practice gap

Embedding EBP is more than just reading journals. There are complex factors about the individual and the context that impact on how we access and apply evidence in our practice. These factors make EBP possibly one of the most challenging change initiatives facing clinicians. This brief overview has served to highlight the principal themes that influence the successful embedding of EBP in clinical practice. There is general consensus that these factors are related to the individual clinicians, their organizational context, the use of specific strategies and agents for change, and aspects of the research evidence. Whilst the evidence from empirical studies has suggested support for each of these effects, it is acknowledged that there remain many unanswered issues regarding the relative interaction of these factors, and the processes by which they influence the use of research knowledge by clinicians. Certainly not all of these barriers will be relevant to all SLTs, in all settings. But an appraisal of relevant personal and local issues will be the optimal starting point for making progress in embedding EBP.

References

Ajzen, I. (1991) The theory of planned behavior. *Organizational Behavior and Human Decision Processes*, 50, 179–211.

Ajzen, I. (2002) Percieved behavioral control, self-efficacy, locus of control, and the theory of planned behaviour. *Journal of Applied Social Psychology*, 32 (4), 665–683.

Baker, M. (1998) Taking the strategy forward. In M. Baker and S. Kirk (eds), *Research and Development for the NHS: Evidence, Evaluation and Effectiveness* (2nd edn). Oxford: Radcliffe Medical Press.

Bannigan, K. and Hooper, L. (2002) How journal clubs can overcome barriers to research utilisation. *British Journal of Therapy and Rehabilitation*, **9** (8), 299–303.

Bonetti, D., Eccles, M., Johnston, M., *et al.* (2005) Guiding the design and selection of interventions to influence the implementation of evidence-based practice: an experimental simulation of a complex intervention trial. *Social Science and Medicine*, **60** (9), 2135–2147.

Brackenbury, T., Burroughs, E. and Hewitt, L.E. (2008) A qualitative examination of current guidelines for evidence-based practice in child language intervention. *Language, Speech and Hearing Services in Schools*, **39**, 78–88.

Closs, S.J. and Lewin, B.J.P. (1998) Perceived barriers to research utilisation: a survey of four therapies. *British Journal of Therapy and Rehabilitation*, **5** (3), 151–155.

Coomarasamy, A. and Khan, S.K. (2004) What is the evidence that postgraduate teaching in evidence based medicine changes anything? A systematic review. *British Medical Journal*, **329**, 1017–1019.

Department of Health (1995) *Methods to promote the implementation of research findings in the NHS – priorities for evaluation. A report to the NHS Central Research and Development Committee.* London: HMSO.

Dopson, S., FitzGerald, L., Ferlie, E., Gabbay, J. and Locock, L. (2002) No magic targets! Changing clinical practice to become more evidence-based. *Health Care Management Review*, **27** (3), 35–47.

Dunn, V., Crichton, N., Roe, B., Seers, K. and Williams, K. (1998) Using research for practice: a UK experience of the BARRIERS scale. *Journal of Advanced Nursing*, **27**, 1203–1210.

Enderby, P. (2004) Evidence-based community rehabilitation: Is it possible? *International Journal of Therapy and Rehabilitation*, **11** (10), 454.

Fish, D. and Coles, C. (1998) *Developing Professional Judgement in Healthcare: Learning Through the Critical Appreciation of Practice.* London: Butterworth Heinemann.

Funk, S.G., Champagne, M.T., Wiese, R.A. and Tornquist, E.M. (1991) Barriers to using research findings in practice: The clinicians' perspective. *Applied Nursing Research*, **4** (2), 90–95.

Gillam, S.L. and Gillam, R.B. (2006) Making evidence-based decisions about child language interventions in schools. *Language, Speech and Hearing Services in Schools*, **37**, 304–315.

Gosling, A.S. and Westbrook, J.I. (2004) Allied health professionals' use of online evidence: A survey of 790 staff working in the Australia public hospital system. *International Journal of Medical Informatics*, **73**, 391–401.

Handy, C. (1999) *Understanding Organisations* (4th edn). London: Penguin.

Ingram, D. (1998) Research-practice relationships in speech-language pathology. *Topics in Language Disorder*, **18** (2), 1–9.

Kajermo, K.N., Nordstrom, G., Krusebrandt, A. and Bjorvell, H. (1998) Barriers to and facilitators of research utilization, as perceived by a group of registered nurses in Sweden. *Journal of Advanced Nursing*, **27**, 798–807.

Kennedy, M. (2002) Principles of assessment. In R. Paul (ed.) *Introduction to Clinical Methods in Communication Disorders.* Baltimore: Brookes.

Kitson, A., Harvey, G. and McCormack, B. (1998) Enabling the implementation of evidence based practice: a conceptual framework. *Quality in Health Care*, 7 (3), 149–158.

Lankshear, A. (2002) An effective survival strategy for evidence-based practice. *British Journal of Therapy and Rehabilitation*, 9 (11), 431–434.

Law, M. and Baum, C. (1998) Evidence-based occupational therapy. *Canadian Journal of Occupational Therapy*, 65 (3), 131–135.

McCleary, L. and Brown, T. (2003) Barriers to paediatric nurses' research utilisation. *Journal of Advanced Nursing*, 42 (4), 364–372.

MacGuire, J.M. (2006) Putting nursing research findings into practice: research utilization as an aspect of the management of change. *Journal of Advanced Nursing*, 53 (1), 65–74.

Metcalfe, C., Lewin, R., Wisher, S., Perry, S., Bannigan, K. and Moffett, J.K. (2001) Barriers to implementing the evidence-base in four NHS therapies: Dieticians, occupational therapists, physiotherapists, speech and language therapists. *Physiotherapy*, 87 (8), 433–441.

Oxman, A.D., Thomson, M.A. and Davis, D.A. (1995) No magic bullets: a systematic review of 102 trials of interventions to improve professional practice. *Canadian Medical Association Journal*, 153, 1423–1431.

Pennington, L. (2001) Attitudes to and use of research in speech and language therapy. *British Journal of Therapy and Rehabilitation*, 8 (10), 375–379.

Pennington, L., Roddam, H., Burton, C., Russell, I., Godfrey, C. and Russell, D. (2005) Promoting research use in speech and language therapy: a cluster randomized controlled trial to compare the clinical effectiveness and costs of two training strategies. *Clinical Rehabilitation*, 19, 387–397.

Pollock, A.S., Legg, L., Langhorne, P. and Sellars, C. (2000) Barriers to achieving evidence-based stroke rehabilitation. *Clinical Rehabilitation*, 14, 611–617.

Roddam, H. (2003) *Promoting the use of research in Speech and Language Therapy departments*. Comite Permanent de Liaison des Orthophonistes-Logopedes de l'Union Europeenne (CPLOL) European Conference, Edinburgh.

Rogers, E.M. (1995) *Diffusion of innovations* (4th edn). New York: The Free Press.

Rosenberg, W. and Donald, A. (1995) Evidence-based medicine: an approach to clinical problem solving. *British Medical Journal*, 310, 1122–1126.

Sackett, D.L., Rosenberg, W.M.C., Gray, J.A.M., Haynes, R.B. and Richardson, W.S. (1996) Evidence-based medicine: What it is and what it isn't. *British Medical Journal*, 312, 71–72.

Stetler, C.B. (2003) The role of the organisation in translating research into evidence-based practice. *Outcomes Management*, 7 (3), 97–103.

Taylor, M. (2000) *Evidence-based Practice for Occupational Therapists*. Oxford: Blackwell Science.

Tse, S., Lloyd, C., Penman, M., King, R. and Bassett, H. (2004) Evidence-based practice and rehabilitation: occupational therapy in Australia and New Zealand experiences. *International Journal of Rehabilitation Research*, 27 (4), 269–274.

Upton, D. (1999) Attitudes towards, and knowledge of, clinical effectiveness in nurses, midwives, practice nurses and health visitors. *Journal of Advanced Nursing*, 29 (4), 885–893.

Upton, D. and Upton, P. (2006) Knowledge and use of evidence-based practice by allied health and health science professionals in the United Kingdom. *Journal of Allied Health*, 35 (3), 127–133.

Vallino-Napoli, L.D. and Reilly, S. (2004) Evidence-based health care: A survey of speech pathology practice. *Advances in Speech and Language Pathology*, **6** (2), 107–112.

van der Gaag, A. and Mowles, C. (2005) Values in professional practice. In C. Anderson and A. van der Gaag (eds), *Speech and Language Therapy: Issues in Professional Practice*. London: Whurr, pp. 10–26.

Veeramah, V. (2004) Utilization of research findings by graduate nurses and midwives. *Journal of Advanced Nursing*, **47** (2), 183–191.

Walker, A., Watson, M., Grimshaw, J. and Bond, C. (2004) Applying the theory of planned behaviour to pharmacists' beliefs and intentions about the treatment of vaginal candidiasis with non-prescription medicines. *Family Practice*, **21**, 670–676.

Walsh, M. (1997) Perceptions of barriers to implementing research. *Nursing Standard*, **11** (19), 34 –37.

Wilks, L. and Boniface, G. (2004) A study of occupational therapists' perceptions of clinical governance. *International Journal of Therapy and Rehabilitation*, **11** (10), 455–460.

Zipoli, R.P. and Kennedy, M. (2005) Evidence-based practice among speech-language pathologists: Attitudes, utilization, and barriers. *American Journal of Speech-Language Pathology*, **14**, 208–220.

Section Two

Developing knowledge and skills for EBP

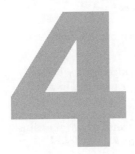

Teaching undergraduates to become critical and effective clinicians

Bea Spek

University Lecturer, Speech and Language Therapy Department,
School of Health Care Studies, Hanze University Groningen,
University of Applied Sciences, The Netherlands

In 2006, a new competence standard, evidence-based practice (EBP), was implemented into the competence-based curriculum for speech and language therapists at Hanze University, Groningen, a city in the northern part of the Netherlands. One of the schools of Hanze University is the School of Health Care Studies, speech and language therapy being one of the departments of this school. The Department of Speech and Language Therapy was founded in 1948 and is with almost 400 students one of the largest departments of speech and language therapy in the Netherlands. The mission of the department of speech and language therapy is to educate students to become critical and socially responsible professionals, and to be a knowledge centre for professionals in the field. The curriculum for speech and language therapy is a 4-year bachelor undergraduate programme. Students are trained in all areas of speech and language therapy. After graduation it is possible to specialize in a particular field. Graduated students obtain the title Bachelor of Health and also a clinical certificate. Some of our students follow a Masters programme that we have in collaboration with the University of Groningen. This takes 1 year extra.

New standards for professional competency

In 2003 the Dutch Association of Logopedics and Phoniatrics (NVLF) updated the professional profile for speech and language therapists (NVLF, 2003). This professional profile was converted into an updated standard competence framework for the education of speech and language therapists in 2004 (Nederlandse Opleidingen Logopedie (SRO), 2005). This was done in collaboration with all seven speech and language educational departments in the Netherlands, the NVLF and representatives of the professional field. This competence framework consists of nine competencies, of which one, competence 2a, deals with providing care. This is shown in Table 4.1.

Table 4.1   Evidence-based practice in the NVLF competency framework

Competency area 1: Prevention, care, training and advice: working with and for clients

Role: Care provider/therapist   Competence 2a. Providing care

The speech and language therapist offers the client(s) speech and language therapy in a professional and sensible manner in order to ease and/or remove the burden of disorders and/or limitations

Sub-competencies	Mastering level 1	Mastering level 2	Mastering level 3	Mastering level 4	Mastering level 5
2a.3 Functions evidence based	I can pose (learning) questions based on a certain problem. I can use information sources effectively and can select the relevant information	I can pose questions following diagnosis and treatment of a case and can use information sources to find relevant research on the subject at hand to use in answering my questions	I can critically judge the validity and practicality of evidence found, even if these are scientific research results. I can create a link between possible solutions and my own practical experiences	I can make choices based on my evidence-based functioning with regard to intervention to individual clients and I can justify and evaluate these choices	I can integrate evidence-based functioning into my own professional functioning

Students are expected to master all nine competencies up to level 5; this means that we must educate undergraduate students to become professionals who can integrate EBP into their clinical practice. We really want students to become critical therapists who have integrated EBP into their own therapeutic acting and thinking. But how to achieve this goal?

The initiative at Hanze University

At Hanze University we use problem-based learning. Students learn via contextualized problem sets and situations. Knowledge, skills and attitudes, which students need to become effective speech and language therapists, are all integrated into clinical cases. Students work on these cases in small groups during their first 10 trimesters. In the last six trimesters, students focus on clinical placements and thesis writing. EBP was a new competence in the updated framework in 2004, which we had to implement in the curriculum. We chose not to teach EBP in a modular form; for example, 1 week of teaching EBP in every year of the curriculum. Instead, we chose to teach EBP in an integrated form; this meant we had to write EBP into all our clinical cases. We did so because we feel that EBP should, as far as possible,

---

Box 4.1   The five steps of evidence-based practice

1.   Asking
Formulating an answerable clinical question
2.   Acquiring
Finding the best available evidence to answer the clinical question
3.   Appraising
Critically evaluating the evidence
4.   Applying
Applying the evidence to your client
5.   Assessing
Monitoring your performance in relation to the evidence

---

be integrated into every professional setting. This would give students the best opportunity to learn not only the principles and skills of EBP but also how to incorporate these skills into their client care. Students should gain an evidence-based attitude. Education in EBP should not only improve knowledge and skills but must actually change behaviour.

Leading in the curriculum are the five steps of EBP (see Box 4.1): asking, acquiring, appraising, applying and assessing, and the five mastering levels of the competence 'EBP' (shown in Table 4.1). It took about 2 years to write all five steps of EBP and all five mastering levels into the curriculum. EBP was implemented step by step, the students of the first year in 2004, the second year in 2005 and the last two years in 2006. The students who started in 2004 are the first students who did the complete cycle of EBP.

EBP in the curriculum

The first year

Every week students get a simple clinical case (see Box 4.2). In these cases the focus is on normal development of speech, language and voice. In tutor groups they focus on formulating their own learning questions around 'what do I need to know to be able to solve this clinical case?' During the week they search for answers to solve their questions and at the end of the week they come together with their tutor and present, justifying their findings. During this first year we do not use the PICO (patient, intervention, comparison, outcome) framework, because students find it difficult just to make good learning questions. Students get a training session with a librarian and a lecturer on how to search the open Internet. Students are familiar with the search engine Google, but most of the time they do not use other search engines like Yahoo and Alta Vista. We teach students how to evaluate a web site. Students must be able to answer questions like: who authored the site?, what is the purpose of the site and the nature of its general content?, and what is the currency of the information? (Nail-Chiwetalu and

---

Box 4.2 Example of a clinical case in the first year

Mrs Andersson is worried about her son Thomas. Mrs Andersson has two children. Emma, 6 years, 6 months old, who attends primary school and is a quick learner. She already reads fluently, and spoke her first words at 11 months. Thomas, 3 years old, is the youngest child. His speech is still poor and sometimes unintelligible. However, his motor skills are excellent; he rides a bike and plays with older children in the crèche. Mrs Andersson wants to know if Thomas' speech is normal for his age or if he needs speech and language therapy.

Task: develop an overview of milestones in normal child development. Focus on motor and speech development.

Bernstein Ratner, 2006). Good information can be obtained on the open Internet, but we teach students where to find it and prompt them to be critical.

We assess basic skills in EBP in a report at the end of the first year. Students have to present an oral paper on an English peer-reviewed study to the whole year group in the lecture room. In this presentation students must show they master the first level of EBP: *I can pose (learning) questions based on a certain problem. I can use information sources effectively and can select the relevant information* (see Table 4.1, above).

The second year

At the beginning of the second year we introduce the five steps of EBP in a lecture (see Box 4.1, above). Students have to practise the first two steps of EBP during the whole year; they must provide every clinical case they study with a clear answerable question, search for evidence in peer-reviewed studies in electronic databases and justify their search strategy and findings (see Box 4.3 for an example case). Questions should be in PICO format: P for patient or problem, I for intervention, C for comparison and O for outcome. To be able to practise the steps of

---

Box 4.3 Example of a clinical case in the second year

Marlies is a little girl 2 years, 1 month old. She suffered from acute meningitis 3 weeks ago, and is not responding to speech and language input according to her parents and doctors. She speaks less than before her illness, and with varying loudness. Hearing tests show sudden deafness. Marlies' previous development was normal. Parental counseling is started, a cochlear implant is considered.

Task: formulate a PICO question and perform a database search. Present and justify your findings in your tutor group.

---

asking and acquiring, students get training sessions with a librarian and the EBP lecturer in formulating PICO questions and searching in electronic databases. In an electronic forum students can post their PICO questions and search strategy and the lecturers on EBP give students feedback.

We assess students' skills in the first two steps of EBP in a written exam by questioning their ability of formulating PICO questions and their knowledge of databases. We use the Fresno test (Ramos *et al.*, 2003) regarding the cycle of EBP, PICO and searching.

The third year

In this year, all five steps of EBP come together: students have already mastered steps one and two, and they now get training sessions in step three: how to appraise the evidence. They must also apply and assess the evidence in a project. During this year, students work in small groups of seven on a project (see Box 4.4 for an example scenario). In this project students have to make an evidence-based guideline. We believe going through this process of making a guideline makes students aware of the importance of evidence-based guidelines and raises actual use of guidelines after graduation. Students get two training sessions on critical appraisal; one using a diagnostic study and one using a therapeutic study. In these sessions we use standardized appraisal instruments of the Dutch Institute for Healthcare Improvement (CBO; www.cbo.nl). Students practise basic statistics in order to be able to make and interpret 2×2 tables. They get training sessions on how to make an observation checklist. Students gather evidence in databases, basic literature and during field work/clinical placements. During the project students can consult the lecturers.

Box 4.4   Example of a clinical case in year 3

Mr Van Boeckholt, MD, works in a small centre for young children with cerebral palsy. Children in this centre also have intellectual disabilities. He notices problems with feeding, like pneumonia and underfeeding. He invites you for an interview in his centre. You are asked to make an evidence-based feeding guideline. This guideline should provide caretakers and parents with useful information about how to prevent the above-mentioned problems. Mr Van Boeckholt is aware of the importance of the social aspect of the feeding situation and wants you to take this into account. One of his questions is how to make optimal use of the communicative abilities of the children. So your guideline should also include advice on how to optimize social aspects in the feeding situation.

Task: Undertake a literature search based on PICO questions. Appraise the evidence found. Visit the centre during a feeding situation and do a careful observation. Use an observation instrument for your visit to the centre. Integrate these findings with the evidence you found in the literature search. Make a guideline for the centre.

We assess students' skills in EBP in an oral exam. In this exam students present and justify their evidence-based guideline. We use the AGREE (Appraisal of Guidelines for Research and Evaluation) appraisal instrument to evaluate their guidelines (The AGREE collaboration, 2001). Students must show that they master level four of EBP: *I can make choices based on my evidence-based functioning with regard to intervention to individual clients and I can justify and evaluate these choices.*

The final phase

The last six trimesters students focus on clinical placements and thesis writing. Students have to provide evidence for their clinical decisions (Box 4.5). In doing so, students go through the whole cycle of EBP. Colleagues in the field act as role models. Their thesis should be based on evidence. Finally, some students participate in research projects or reviews with lecturers.

Box 4.5   Example of a clinical question during external placements in the last six trimesters

A few weeks ago, Mrs Constantine, a speech and language therapist, attended an education workshop on non-speech oral motor therapy. In this therapy a Forcescale and a myoscanner are used to measure lip strength and tongue strength. Mrs Constantine wonders if these measures are reliable and valid.

   Task: Do a literature search on diagnostic instruments used in non-speech oral motor therapy. Perform a pilot study on the inter-rater reliability and validity of these instruments. Integrate these findings with the evidence you found in the literature search. Write a recommendation to Mrs Constantine about your findings.

Challenges to developing and implementing an evidence-focused curriculum

The quality of the evidence

As expected, it is quite a challenge for students to provide evidence for every clinical case they work on. What to do with cases on which there is no evidence available or where evidence is of low quality? Our profession is relatively young and has a limited research tradition (Dodd, 2007). There are not many randomized control trials or systematic reviews and the ones found are not very encouraging. In some diagnostic categories you do not find any evidence at all. We have to teach students how to deal with this. We always emphasize that EBP is founded on three pillars: scientific evidence, therapeutic skills and clients' values and preferences. It is not all about research evidence and sometimes you have to rely on expert opinions or best practices.

The role of statistics

Critical appraisal appears to be challenging because of difficulties undergraduate students are facing with statistics. We feel that even with only basic statistic skills, students can actually appraise scientific research papers by just using the right tools and their own critical mind. It is possible to teach undergraduates the meaning of effect measures like absolute benefit increase, number needed to treat, relative risk reduction and so on. We also teach our students diagnostic measurement concepts like specificity, sensitivity, positive predictive value and negative predictive value. In our experience even weaker students are able to cope with these concepts. Even without doing any research it is possible to appraise scientific evidence.

Controversy among lecturers

Although the definition of EBP is agreed upon world-wide: *the conscientious, explicit and judicious use of current best evidence in making decisions about the care of individual patients* (Sackett *et al.*, 1997), lecturers questioned the meaning of this. Do students have to provide every clinical case with evidence, would this not take too much of their time? Should we develop clinical cases on which we know there is evidence, and what to do then with other clinical cases, should we just skip them? Not all lecturers welcome EBP; some lecturers feel EBP is just a passing phase, while others see EBP as a great opportunity to improve the quality of speech and language therapy. Not all lecturers are educated in EBP and fear it might be too difficult for them. There was discussion about the place EBP should have. We feel the School of Health Care Studies has an important role in this, the school should reflect the relevance of EBP. So we issued a standard on EBP for all departments of the School of Health Care Studies. In this standard, criteria are formulated for every step in EBP. All departments, including Physiotherapy, Nutrition and Dietetics, Oral Hygiene, Medical Imaging and Radiation Oncology, and Speech and Language Therapy, have to adhere to this standard. Every year we organize a small conference on EBP for all lecturers of the School of Healthcare Studies. New colleagues are trained in EBP and lecturers in EBP act as contact point for every lecturer.

Colleagues in the field

Most students are eager to master all the competencies, and during their external placements, they expect to be able to put their competencies into practice. However, in the field of speech and language therapy, interest in EBP is relatively young. Most speech and language therapists first consult colleagues while seeking information, followed by textbooks, continuing education workshops and the open Internet (Nail-Chiwetalu and Bernstein Ratner, 2006). They do not always seek information in peer-reviewed publications; they may not even have access to these resources. So, a gap exists between the knowledge and skills of our students, and the actual clinical decision-making process by professionals in the field. Students might become frustrated if they do not get the opportunity to use EBP skills in their placements. Once a year free training sessions on EBP are provided for colleagues in the field. In 2008 a journal club for students, lecturers and colleagues in the field started. Access to full text resources is a great problem for our colleagues, so we encourage them to make use of the students when searching for evidence. In collaboration with all educational institutions for speech and language therapy in the Netherlands, we produce a monthly column in the *Dutch Journal for Logopedics and Phoniatrics*, in which we appraise research studies (Spek and de Beer, 2007).

Reflection

We see in our students, lecturers and colleagues in the field a growing awareness that EBP is important for our profession. There is a change from seeing EBP as a threat to seeing it as an opportunity to improve the quality of speech and language therapy. Attitudes are actually changing. However, changing of behaviour takes a lot of time and patience.

When teaching EBP in the profession of speech and language therapy, it is important to encourage students to understand the three pillars of EBP being scientific evidence, therapeutic skills and clients' values and preferences. The focus should not only be on the role of scientific evidence. It is also important to take your time and not to expect too much. EBP is not too difficult for undergraduate students, it really is possible to teach undergraduates to become critical therapists who have integrated EBP into their own therapeutic acting and thinking. Creating lifelong learners is a key aim. The most important thing is to realize that EBP is not a threat but that it is a great opportunity for our profession.

Acknowledgements

Ellen de Wit, MSc and Inge Wijkamp, MSc for their helpful suggestions on this chapter.

References

Dodd, B. (2007) EBP and speech-language pathology: Strength, weaknesses, opportunities and threats. *Folia Phoniatrica et Logopaedica*, 59, 118–129.

Nail-Chiwetalu, B.J. and Bernstein Ratner, N. (2006) Information literacy for speech-language pathologists: A key to EBP. *Language, Speech and Hearing Services in Schools*, 37 (7), 157–167.

Nederlandse Opleidingen Logopedie (SRO) (2005) *Compass Competency Profile Speech and Language Therapy Student* (1st edn). Drukkerij SchrijenLippertzHuntjens.

Nederlandse Vereniging voor Logopedie en Foniatrie (2003) *Beroepsprofiel logopedist*. Gouda: NVLF.

Ramos, K.D., Schafer, S. and Tracz, S.M. (2003) Validation of the Fresno test of competence in evidence-based medicine. *British Medical Journal*, 326 (7384), 319–321.

Sackett, D.L., Richardson, W.S., Rosenberg, W.M.C. and Haynes, R.B. (1997) *Evidence-based medicine: How to practice and teach EBM*. London: Churchill Livingstone.

Spek, B. and de Beer, J. (2007) Rubriek evidence-based logopedie. *Logopedie en foniatrie*, **79** (3), 78–79.

The AGREE collaboration (2001) Appraisal of Guidelines for Research and Evaluation (AGREE) instrument. Retrieved 14 July 2008, from www.agreecollaboration.org

Promoting clinical effectiveness with postgraduate students

Paula Leslie[1] and James L. Coyle[2]

[1]Associate Professor, Department of Communication Science
and Disorders, University of Pittsburgh, USA
[2]Assistant Professor, Department of Communication Science
and Disorders, University of Pittsburgh, USA

Standard US speech and language therapy/therapist (SLT) graduate programmes are being increasingly challenged in successfully preparing students with the knowledge and skills needed to practise as professionals especially in medical SLT settings. Modern healthcare provision has to be evidence-based but many clinicians struggle to find the evidence, evaluate it, produce it, or disseminate it. Wherever a professional is on the clinician-researcher continuum they need basic research skills. Our roles within the Department of Communication Science and Disorders (CSD) at the University of Pittsburgh, as well as our clinical backgrounds in SLT in the US and the UK, have given us an interest in these issues. We have both been involved in the development of a Doctor of Clinical Science degree at the University of Pittsburgh. In this chapter we will describe how this new degree programme supports the development of clinical effectiveness in our students.

Background: SLT training in the US

The American higher educational system is organized into undergraduate and graduate-level programmes. Students graduating from high schools enter universities and colleges, earning a Bachelor's degree usually in four years of study. Students may then apply to graduate school. Graduate level education includes programmes culminating in the Master of Arts or Master of Science degrees in most disciplines, and is from one to three years duration. Communication sciences and disorders programmes are usually two years in length. Since the 1930s 'speech therapists' with a four year Bachelor's degree in Communication Disorders were certified to provide therapeutic services to children and adults with speech, language, and voice problems. In 1965 in recognition of the growth in the breadth and depth of populations served, the educational standards for entry level certification were raised to a Master's degree: typically a two year post-Bachelor's graduate degree (Shames and Anderson, 2002).

In the current system in the US there are two distinct foci of clinical practice: medical and educational SLT (Lubinski and Frattali, 1994). There are slightly more SLTs employed by the nation's public school systems than healthcare. SLTs are front-line providers of consultative, diagnostic, and intervention services to adults and children with a wide range of medical conditions including dysphagia services.

In order to complete the requirements to gain the clinical certificate (CCC-SLP) from the American Speech and Hearing Association (ASHA), which is needed to practise as an SLT, students must sit an exam and undertake a supervised Clinical Fellowship once they complete their Master's degree. This fellowship is a probationary period when the clinical fellow receives extra supervision and periodic, documented mentoring.

Medical SLTs: The need to develop evidence-based clinical experts

The expansion of the scope of practice of the SLT has generated perhaps the most important pressure on the field. In the last twenty years we have seen additions to the SLT role with management in adults and children including oropharyngeal dysphagia. Dysphagia now makes up the majority of the caseload for more than 40% of American SLTs. These SLTs have assumed the rehabilitation of upper aerodigestive tract function in tracheotomized and ventilator-dependent patients, and the assessment and treatment of head and neck trauma associated with military events. Videofluoroscopy and endoscopy have become essential diagnostic tools employed exclusively by the SLT in evaluation of the head and neck.

Medical SLTs work as part of an interdisciplinary team with physicians and other medical professionals. They must have advanced medical knowledge and use complex instrumentation to differentially diagnose and treat patients with communication, cognitive and swallowing disorders. Expert clinical leaders must be developed who are adept at managing the external and internal pressures of the modern health care system and its rapidly changing landscape. To address this need the Communication Science and Disorders Department at the University of Pittsburgh embarked on a plan to create a unique professional doctorate in Medical Speech Language Pathology. This Doctor of Clinical Science degree (CScD) would supplement the entry level Master's degree. The CScD was designed primarily for SLTs wishing to develop high level clinical specialization, expertise, and leadership in the medical setting.

Unlike the Doctor of Philosophy (PhD) degree where training is focused on research, the CScD is a full-time programme that prepares clinically advanced SLTs. Such professionals apply evidenced-based diagnostic and therapeutic methods to healthcare. Education is provided through a combination of classroom instruction, case-based learning, and multidisciplinary clinical rotations at state of the art primary care, acute and rehabilitation medical centres. Students work closely with clinical experts, accomplished mentors and researchers in communication science and disorders. Clinical specialization is possible depending on the student's interest, educational background and experience level.

Developing the Doctor of Clinical Science degree programme

As with any new programme a case for the need for such an initiative had to be made to the University. This included the rationale for the programme, the desired outcomes and a structure for its delivery. Surveys of existing students and practising clinicians were taken to gauge potential future interest and potential employers such as the federally funded Veteran's Affairs Health System were consulted.

Was the idea unique to the US? When the programme was first conceived it was presumed that no one had experience in such clinical and academic education at post qualification level. It is quite a challenge to design and implement the first of a type. A strength of the CSD department at Pittsburgh is the solid link between clinic and classroom from a teaching perspective. This clinic–classroom link is further supported by several members of the department who are highly respected in academic circles and who also carry external clinical caseloads. Although working in the UK (Paula) and the USA (James), we met through a mutual interest in dysphagia and evidence-based practice (EBP). We found that we were both implementing a similar programme in our own countries.

When the designs and rationales behind the UK and US programmes were studied, the overlap was astonishing – in fundamental ethos and in practicalities. What this suggests is that the need for post-qualification and EBP education is a global concern. Clearly, some issues that face SLT professionals are without borders, and the need for clinicians to be trained in EBP is one issue that applies equally well across countries. Independently of each other the CScD and the UK Research Masters grew from an identified clinician need and a professional leap was made. Paula Leslie is now in Pittsburgh helping to implement the US programme.

The Clinical Doctorate at Pittsburgh

The fundamental areas covered in the Pittsburgh Clinical Doctorate programme are highlighted in Box 5.1.

We wanted clinicians to leave the programme prepared for independence, leadership, excellence in clinical practice, and able to undertake clinical teaching positions in universities. A cornerstone of the programme is extensive reading and critical evaluation of literature. The focus on EBP takes place throughout the course.

Tiered entry points

These are from post-Bachelor to post-Doctoral students and returning licensed clinicians. We wanted to attract students across a range of life experiences so we created a tiered entry system. People can enter the programme at different stages: for example, post-Bachelor's degrees up to PhD researchers and practising clinicians with years of experience. Students entering with an appropriate Bachelor's degree can meet Master's entry-level requirements during the first two years of the CScD programme. Practising clinicians (with Master's degree and CCC-SLP) can enter the course for Years 3–5; such students have considerable clinical experience which can be shared as a fantastic learning resource.

Box 5.1   Fundamental areas covered in the Clinical Doctorate programme

Advanced clinical practice: including the interplay of ethics and evidence in complex decision making; for example, students attend clinical decision making meetings both within and outside of the SLT profession and report back on the process as well as the content.

EBP: this includes extensive reading and critical appraisal of the literature to underpin all assignments, as well as specific teaching about research methods.

Leadership skills: students attend a course in leadership relevant to their own practice, so it might be in the business school or through a multidisciplinary developmental delay team.

Interdisciplinary issues: approximately 25% of the programme requires students to choose courses outside of CSD so they participate in classes with students from the professions that we work with clinically.

Professional dissemination of information: students learn the importance of the audience/readership perspective in oral presentations and written papers as well as the mechanics of how to do both.

Mentored externships

From the third year of the course onwards, students work clinically for 50% of the week. This clinical work takes place in an adult or paediatric medical SLT setting such as acute or rehabilitation hospitals, or special school setting. The university identifies and works with potential employers to develop these posts and to ensure that there is some flexibility for students, as the academic timetable can vary. The students are paid the *pro rata* salary for the post, which helps to offset educational and living costs. Whilst in these clinical posts the students are 'mentored' by members of the CSD department at the university. The term 'clinical mentored experience' is used to differentiate the clinical posts that the students hold from posts that are not linked to the university. The term also differentiates the more usual clinical 'placement' that a precertification student would hold. The mentored externships are assessed using case presentations, reflective learning journals and targets created each semester between the students and their particular mentors. The mentors are rotated among students each year, to encourage development across a range of fields and perspectives.

Customized education

Students entering in the third year of the course can choose to focus many aspects of their studies to match their interests and the requirements of their jobs. For example, although courses are required in anatomy, students can choose to take an adult head and neck anatomy course or a paediatric craniofacial course to qualify. Courses can also be balanced around the clinical mentored experience requirements outlined above.

Research methods education

As noted in Box 5.1, EBP is one of the fundamental areas of the CScD course. It is important to develop knowledge that enables clinicians to find and evaluate evidence to support their clinical practice. Teaching methods aim to develop skills in all areas from the outset. All assignments are supported by critical appraisal of the literature and presented in written and oral media, matching information dissemination methods in the real world.

Oral presentation focus

Giving students experience with oral presentations develops a transferable, essential skill and allows the sharing of a significant body of experience. Oral presentations allow us to share the learning that we could not do from say, twenty essays. As noted in Box 5.1 we focus on professional dissemination of information. Students participate in medical case conferences and present to multidisciplinary teams. Assignments are clinically focused and individually tailored which contributes to the development of knowledge in the student's clinical workplace. Sharing this work allows students and instructors to access the most up-to-date body of evidence in medical SLT.

Developing highly skilled, evidence-based clinicians: impact of the CScD course

In the US the profession has yet to develop universal recognition of the need for a Clinical Doctorate such as we offer at the University of Pittsburgh. Yet, there is widespread recognition that the breadth and depth of knowledge necessary to effectively practise as an SLT in modern tertiary medical and trauma centres far exceeds the content provided in traditional entry level education. It is unlikely that the Clinical Doctorate will ever be necessary for ordinary practice in most settings. In the competitive, rapidly evolving and multidimensional modern medical setting the need for such education is already established. The ability of cutting edge, progressive academic programmes to recognize and fulfil the need for clinical experts and leaders, is essential for the future of the SLT profession in the medical setting.

The first graduates from our programme should complete their studies in 2010. Currently we have students entering at Year 1 and 3. Some are entering Year 3 straight from a Master's programme and must complete their clinical fellowship. Other students are entering the Year 3 with their clinical licence and many years of experience.

The CScD course focuses on creating experts and leaders in the application of evidence based practice. Students take these skills and knowledge out into the clinical world. There is often a gap between what students are taught in the classroom and what clinicians are doing in practice. Sometimes this is a learning process for the students and sometimes for the clinical supervisor. When managed well it is mutually beneficial to both sides: learning about the latest evidence and the integration with informed clinical experience. The feedback from students suggests that they find the EBP focus to be important to developing their leadership skills, for example, one wrote:

EBP lacked during my graduate programme. I want to educate and apply EBP into our field, which starts from the beginning as a student ... I learned directly from inspiring, dynamic academic professors in this field. I want to impart the knowledge and skills (particularly as a consumer of research and to appraise the literature clinically) they taught me to future students. (Clinically licensed SLT who has worked for five years prior to beginning the CScD).

Students also report the benefits of having access to courses outside of the areas covered in traditional SLT courses. One student who began the course straight after completing her Master's in SLT, reported:

One of the strengths of the programme is that it encourages students to take courses outside of the field of speech-language pathology. Last year, I took gross anatomy and physiology courses with first-year dental students. I received hands-on experience with prosection and dissection of cadavers. I now can read medical charts with a better understanding of my patient's injuries and how that can impact communication, swallowing and cognition.

Some of the students from Year 3 and above act as clinical supervisors of students who are just beginning the course (Years 1 and 2). We have included education in clinical supervision and this dual role of supervisor and student is investigated by self reflected learning journals completed by all students. By ensuring that presentations and some seminars are attended by students in all years of the programme, the senior students (who are clinically active) can form role models for the more junior students. One of the supervising students reflected on this, writing:

In some ways I'm 'in-between' the experts (my mentors and professors) and the students. What I learn from my mentoring and classes eventually trickles down to how and what I teach my students. In a way, this is a preview of what I think one of the goals of the CScD should be, i.e. creating clinicians who are able to digest and translate information from experts to other clinicians and students. (Clinically licensed SLT who has worked for more than fifteen years prior to beginning the CScD).

One of the main assessments of the mentored externships involves presentation of cases and medical conditions to different types of audience such as medical case conferences, multidisciplinary teams, and local caregiver support groups. This models EBP for other SLTs, healthcare professionals and the public. All CScD students from Years 1 to 5 attend these together with teaching staff. This encourages sharing of information and the junior students can see where they are headed.

Reflections on the CScD course

The main challenges to the programme are finding appropriate clinical posts, funding for students for three–five years of study, and the current restriction that students must attend study in Pittsburgh. We are investigating ways to deliver some of the curriculum at a distance and online whilst retaining the integrity of the programme (e.g. sharing of education and experiences between all students, face to face interaction between the expert clinical educators and the students). We are getting applications from overseas students, and other institutes in the US are asking for advice on how to set up such a programme indicating that the programme will be sustainable in the long term.

There is a need for medical SLTs and others interested in advanced clinical thinking skills to receive further education. This is a starting point to addressing the need of the expanding field of knowledge and skills required for the successful practice of the SLT profession. There is clearly broad international interest in furthering our profession's clinical–academic education. The Pittsburgh programme is one such model to ensure that medical SLTs become highly skilled evidence-based practitioners.

References

Lubinski, R. and Frattali, C. (eds). (1994) *Professional Issues in Speech-Language Pathology and Audiology*. San Diego: Singular.

Shames, G. and Anderson, N. (2002) *Human Communication Disorders*. Boston: Allyn & Bacon.

Clinical effectiveness: not just a journal club

Satty Boyes[1] and Gina Sutcliffe[2]

[1]Manager, Speech and Language Therapy Department,
Salford Primary Care Trust, UK
[2]Senior Speech and Language Therapist, Speech and Language Therapy
Department, Salford Primary Care Trust, UK

This chapter describes an approach taken by a service in a large UK adult teaching hospital with a strong research culture, to implement a structured approach to clinical effectiveness. The first section explores how research appraisal contributed to the wider concept of clinical effectiveness and describes the leadership and quality improvement philosophy that has underpinned the initiative. The latter part of the chapter describes the process undertaken and some of the practicalities that have been considered in introducing our approach to clinical effectiveness.

Satty Boyes manages the service. She completed her Masters degree in a quality-management related topic. This learning has framed the philosophy of the approach developed, linking it clearly to quality and the concept of continuous improvement. As a senior clinician, Gina Sutcliffe has utilized her skills in research, development and project management to translate our shared vision into a practical model for the service to use.

Underpinning philosophy

Services are accountable to deliver the best available interventions to the population they serve within the constraints of the resources available to them. In order to achieve this, clinicians need to integrate evidence into their decision-making about interventions to ensure that the services they develop and deliver are clinically effective. Furthermore, in order to expand services and attract additional resources, clinicians must be able to demonstrate benefits to clients and other professionals. Research appraisal is therefore a key element of clinical effectiveness.

Traditionally, a large focus has been placed on critical appraisal and this has prompted the emergence of many journal clubs. Our own experiences of journal clubs have highlighted many issues that hinder success. These include: relevance of the papers being studied to the service; knowledge and skills of the attendees in carrying out critical appraisal; time to develop skills within the whole team; the departmental culture; and the leadership responsibility taken by the manager. The literature has also highlighted common barriers to successful evidence-based journal clubs including: access to library resources and the skills to use them; confidence in critical appraisal and access to relevant training; lack of opportunity to discuss research evidence with colleagues (Bourne *et al.*, 2007). Additionally, even when journal club approaches have been successful in supporting critical appraisal skills, these skills represent only one element of evidence-based practice (EBP), since learning from research and implementing best practice need to be embedded within the context of the whole service. Focusing on research appraisal alone does not address the need to integrate learning into service delivery and quality improvement.

We felt that there were a number of key factors which would help to promote the success of launching any form of journal club for increasing clinical effectiveness. First, strong leadership would be crucial, with the speech and language therapy (SLT) manager taking responsibility for actively promoting a culture that would allow quality and clinical effectiveness to thrive. We also recognized that there was a need to ensure that any projects / improvements were planned within the context of the wider organizational goals and their impact was carefully measured. The SLT service manager would need to take responsibility for translating the aims of the organization and the wider health service into service level priorities, which would allow the rest of the team to focus on service-oriented objectives and to be able to prioritize these effectively. We hoped that this would promote a genuine sense of team ownership of this initiative, with everyone sharing a common understanding of our philosophy, vision and aims. Other published studies (including Gilbody, 1996) indicated that this team philosophy might not only contribute to clinical effectiveness but could also support members to develop the confidence to professionally challenge and question practice, and in turn drive the identification of topics and areas in the service that required review to consolidate best practice, and to identify areas for service improvement.

We looked for a framework that would help us to make a strategic plan to achieve these goals. A 'plan, do, check, act' (PDCA) cycle is commonly used to support quality improvement (Deming, 1992) and we decided to use this model to describe the process we would undertake to support clinical effectiveness. Figure 6.1 summarizes the elements we felt to be essential and how these are linked.

The PDCA cycle helped us to consider the key concepts of continuous quality improvement and systems thinking. Systems thinking theory recognizes that any process we undertake has many different parts. None of these operate in isolation and the outcome of a process is dependent on how the different parts interact. Therefore if we want a process to be successful, we need to ensure that all the elements required are structured and interact in a way to maximize the end results. We believe that understanding these concepts has helped us to develop our systematic approach to service improvement and hence to clinical effectiveness; since without implementing a holistic approach to EBP, the quality of the service – and more importantly, the benefits to the client – could not be fully realized.

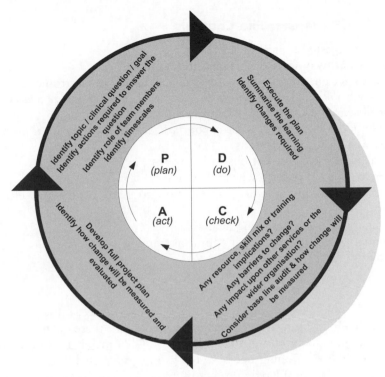

Figure 6.1   Plan, do, check, act (PDCA) cycle (Deming, 1992).

The Clinical Effectiveness Group

Development of the group

On careful consideration of the definition of EBP and the pitfalls experienced previously, a new group was developed called the Clinical Effectiveness Group (CEG). The CEG was introduced as a group with a clear focus on identifying potential research areas of interest and processing these in a positive way, encompassing all aspects of clinical effectiveness, not just critical appraisal. Members were informed that this would be a forum to which they could bring their ideas and clinical queries to a group of people with a shared interest in investigating relevant topics. A CEG master file was developed containing all relevant information so that it was at members' fingertips (Box 6.1).

When the initiative was introduced, staff were invited to complete a questionnaire to indicate their level of confidence in areas relating to formulating research questions, literature searching, critical appraisal and audit. It was anticipated that staff would be more candid in their responses if the questionnaires were submitted anonymously. Training was organized for members of the group to target areas of reduced confidence. For example, the organization's research and development department agreed to provide training in formulating a research question. The library service agreed to complete literature searches and source papers for the

---

Box 6.1   CEG Master File Contents

- List of suggested topics for CEG
- Process pathway for CEG (shown in Figure 6.2)
- How to get an Athens password to enable access to electronic resources
- Library booklet: *A Brief Guide to Carrying out a Literature Search*
- List of search engines (e.g. Cochrane Library, PubMed)
- Guide: *How to access the list of journals available in the local area* (hard copy and electronic versions)
- Phone numbers and locations of librarians
- Copy of journal order forms and summary of process and cost
- Summary of copyright laws in relation to hard copies and electronic journals
- Summary of library training available
- Summary of EBP and critical appraisal training
- Copy of critical appraisal tools

---

group in a timely fashion. Agreements were made with these agencies as to how they could support the group in the longer term. CEG members were encouraged to identify their own training needs as the group progressed, allowing emerging training needs to be considered and met in areas such as change management.

CEG process

A process pathway for clinical effectiveness was developed (Figure 6.2) and included in the CEG manual. The first step in this pathway was the identification of suitable questions. Clinicians were asked to note down topics they questioned in their mind, whether this be during day to day working, or stimulated through meetings and courses. Topics might be stimulated through phrases like 'if I had time, I'd look into ...' or 'I think we should be ...'. Issues relating to both individual client groups and larger service delivery questions were encouraged. In this way, specific questions were raised for investigation and recorded at the front of the CEG file for group discussion and possible selection for future processing. Compared to earlier journal clubs which were centred on critical appraisal of single research articles, the CEG was goal oriented, with a focus very much on a team approach to answering the research questions.

As a topic was completed, the end of that meeting was used to select the new topic and agree the research question appropriate to this. The topics were varied to allow different clinical areas of interest to be catered for over the course of time. A member of the team was assigned to organize each literature search. This person was changed each time in order to share the preparation work load between the group members. They were often selected as they had proposed the topic for processing by the group or had the strongest interest in that area. Their role was to contact the library with the agreed research question, to request a literature search summary, select appropriate papers from the summary and request a full copy of these papers for the group. Papers were then screened for length and dis-

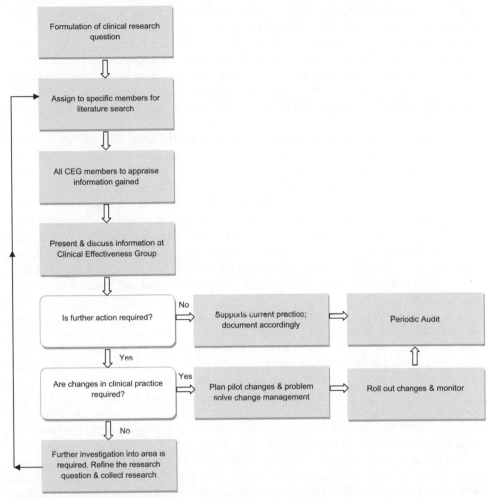

Figure 6.2 Process pathway for clinical effectiveness (Sutcliffe, 2008).

tributed evenly throughout the group two weeks before the next meeting with a copy of the agreed research question as a guide. At least two people were assigned to read each paper to stimulate discussion within the group, increase the reliability of the appraisal carried out and provide support for those assigned more difficult papers. Copies of critical appraisal tools were available for the group to use throughout this process.

At the next meeting, group members were reminded of the research question and invited to contribute a verbal summary of each of the papers they appraised. Points for discussion were noted throughout by the CEG leader and raised at appropriate times to stimulate discussion and clarify the outcomes to be agreed for that meeting. Following the meeting, the final outcomes were e-mailed to the group inviting comments for alterations to wording or content within one week. These outcome sheets were then dated and recorded in the completed topics file for future reference.

The aim was to pursue a topic until a satisfactory outcome was achieved, not to abandon topics part way through the process. A broad range of research evidence was included, from single case studies to large randomized control studies, with the strengths and weaknesses of the methodology being considered by the group during discussion. If poor methodology of the research studied meant the question could not be answered, a refined question would be agreed, further evidence searched for or a date set to revisit the topic at an appropriate time in the future.

The outcome of the CEG process depended on the question. In some cases, further areas of interest were added to the list for future processing. In others, we made plans for clinical audits of current practice and agreed action plans to pilot clinical changes required in line with new evidence. An appropriate member of the CEG was assigned to oversee the pilot of the changes depending upon their area of experience and these were included within staff appraisal objectives as appropriate. Full discussions of the impact these changes may have upon other professionals and services took place. Depending upon the proposed changes, these discussions have included considerations of the boundaries of the SLT role, training of others in our reasoning for the proposed changes in practice and the potential resource implications.

Our group leader was a senior SLT. This person was selected based on having the skills required to lead the CEG and guide research-based discussions, rather than on clinical seniority. The leader was not viewed as an 'expert' in EBP but someone to guide and chair the meetings. Every effort was made to retain a non-judgemental atmosphere, to invite equal participation from members with varying degrees of experience in different clinical areas and allow them to express their views freely. Small group work or work in pairs was preferred to enforce the feeling of shared responsibility and retain a team approach. This supported members to build confidence in their participation.

The practical issues of frequency and duration of groups took time to agree. Initial plans to hold the meetings 'as required' were not successful and so dates were agreed every 8 weeks. Only one topic was processed at a time, most of which were completed within one or two meetings; however larger topics took more time to process. Recording clear outcomes assisted the group in being able to complete topics in a time efficient manner. It was recognized that should clear outcomes not be agreed, some topics had potential to be processed indefinitely which would not be good use of time and would limit the success of the group. Topics were agreed as 'completed' when a satisfactory level of evidence was collated in response to the research question. However, a date was sometimes agreed to revisit some 'completed' topics with the aim of monitoring potential future evidence. Completed topics were stored as a pack of evidence with a front sheet summarizing the research question, points learned, difficulties encountered and the outcome/action plan.

No actual agreement was made that the meetings were to be a high priority but as interest grew in the topics being processed, commitment developed. Members were requested to send their contribution if they were unable to attend meetings, to allow progress of the topics within the group in their absence.

Information from a variety of sources was shared during the meetings including course information, new clinical guidelines or revision of existing clinical guidelines to allow further investigation of areas and/or actions plans to be formulated in relation to these.

Reflections on the impact of the CEG

Previous journal clubs, focusing on critical appraisal alone, often achieved very little from a clinical perspective. The common methodological problems in the SLT literature, for example small study design, author bias and small sample size, were encountered on a frequent basis and led to unproductive meetings. Approaching the evidence in this way overlooked the value of smaller scale research, as no clinical change could be justified on one of these studies alone. It did not allow these studies to be viewed as a valuable part of a hierarchy of evidence for that clinical area. In addition, clinicians would visibly bristle at the prospect of being involved in critical appraisal and very few clinicians were brave enough to nominate themselves as journal club organizer.

This often led to a series of cancelled meetings and eventual dissolution of groups as clinicians justified their time being spent better elsewhere. Clearly, this approach was lacking in many ways.

So far, the CEG has achieved an evidence base for decisions regarding clinical management for specific client groups and provided support for current practice. It has expanded knowledge through reading and facilitated improved consistency in the clinical knowledge of the members. Members have reported a greater confidence in the topics studied and report that they are able to justify their clinical decision-making more clearly. When reviews have supported current clinical practice, members have been encouraged to engage in EBP further, as it has strengthened the link between research and clinical practice.

Currently, our group consists of SLTs only. However, it would be anticipated that a CEG could comprise members from different disciplines, with the primary requisite being a shared interest in a particular area and a willingness to engage in the clinical questions raised by other group members. Members are able to broaden their own knowledge and skills but are also reassured that a future topic of their choice will receive that depth of attention from the group. This brings a clinical value to the group that a single clinician could never achieve in isolation. We have been delighted that the CEG model has started to be used as an example of good practice within our organization. The Trust are considering rolling out the model to other departments, to be led by designated Team Knowledge Officers, as part of a project to encourage Trust-wide use of EBP.

To date, we have not experienced any resistance to change from within the SLT department or from other members of staff. However, we are aware that resistance may raise itself as an issue in the future. Larger scale changes to practice that may be raised by CEG topics may impact upon other health professionals' roles or perception of our role, and this may raise potential areas of conflict. Similarly, the team may need to implement changes that require a substantial amount of resources to execute in the broader context of the organization. We anticipate that our more inclusive approach to gathering and appraising evidence will provide a comprehensive rationale for the changes to practice that we need to implement.

Changes in membership of the CEG have been managed carefully. The CEG manual provides a useful overview and guide for the training of new members of staff joining the group. New members have been paired with existing members during their first few attendances, to support their skills and confidence when contributing. We have found that this approach works well with all levels of staff by providing support in the practical aspects of CEG participation such as leading a literature search and also encouraging active participation within the group discussions without fear of criticism.

Implementation of the CEG has required a high level of commitment to clinical effectiveness among clinicians and managers in our team. Key to our approach was a need to ensure we developed a holistic and systematic model that related not only to the topics being appraised but also to the wider quality and service improvement agendas. Our strong team commitment to being evidence-based clinicians is anticipated to be the driving force that will support a productive and sustainable CEG.

Acknowledgements

The authors would like to thank Dr James Boyes for formatting the figures for this chapter.

References

Bourne, J.A., Dziedzic, K., Morris, S.J., Jones, P.W. and Sim, J. (2007) Survey of the perceived professional, educational and personal needs of physiotherapists in primary care and community settings. *Health and Social Care in the Community*, 15 (3), 231–237.

Deming, W.E. (1992) *Out of the Crisis* (18th edn). Cambridge: Cambridge University Press.

Gilbody, S. (1996) Evidence-based medicine: an improved format for journal clubs. *Psychiatric Bulletin*, 20, 673–675.

Sutcliffe, G. (2008) Process pathway for clinical effectiveness. Unpublished resource created in the Salford PCT Adult Speech and Language Therapy Department.

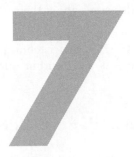

Using evidence-based practice in supervision

Hannah Crawford

Consultant Speech and Language Therapist,
Tees, Esk and Wear Valleys NHS Trust, UK

I am a speech and language therapist (SLT) based in County Durham (UK) specializing in dysphagia in adults with learning disabilities. I work for an NHS trust and carry responsibility for the development and implementation of the dysphagia service to adults with learning disability across the trust. This includes the clinical supervision of all of the SLTs working for the trust. I have additional roles as a tutor on Manchester Metropolitan University's Advanced Dysphagia course, and as co-chair of the ALD Dysphagia UK group, whose aim is to facilitate the sharing and development of good practice and clinical research in this area.

The drive to increase clinicians' engagement with patient-centred, evidence-based practice (EBP) has never been more pressing. There is pressure from managers and commissioners/purchasers of services to prove that what we do works for patients. We have a professional responsibility to measure the effectiveness of what we do. For the benefit of our patients we need to investigate what works and what doesn't. We should strive to question, evaluate, and develop our practice in a systematic way. We should then share and reflect on what works and what doesn't, thereby increasing the evidence that guides our practice. Clinical supervision is one means of achieving these aims. Within our SLT department, supervision is one of the mechanisms we use for evaluating and developing our practice in an evidence-based way.

The Royal College of Speech and Language Therapists (RCSLT) advises that all SLTs should access clinical supervision at least every 12 weeks (RCSLT, 2006). RCSLT state that clinical supervision can 'assist the practitioner in relating practice to theory and theory to practice (p. 104) … [and] create a learning environment which promotes critical reflective practice' (p. 105). This clearly resonates with the model of EBP proposed by Sackett *et al.* (1996), who stated that:

> the practice of evidence-based medicine means integrating individual clinical
> expertise with the best available external clinical evidence … and in the more
> thoughtful identification and compassionate use of individual patients'

predicaments, rights, and preferences in making clinical decisions about their care (p. 71).

This 'triad' of evidence-based medicine (Sackett *et al.*, 1997) – that is clinical experience, best available evidence and patient preference – is used within our department to frame case discussions in supervision.

Development of supervision systems in our department

Within our Trust, there has always been a strong focus on supervision, with the SLT manager believing strongly in its value in terms of clinical support and development. There is a strong belief that this support and development is crucial for SLTs, in terms of their clinical competence and confidence, and benefits the patients by ensuring robust, up to date and appropriate intervention.

I have been working in a clinical leadership position for eight years. On taking up this post, one of the requirements was to roll out specific clinical supervision in dysphagia. I aimed to follow the existing structures of individual supervision, where clinicians can air individual issues and concerns, and discuss details of particular clinical cases, as well as group supervision, where ideas and concerns can be shared and others can contribute and learn.

The evidence that guided the development of the dysphagia supervision systems included:

- RCSLT guidance on regularity of supervision (RCSLT, 2006)
- the NHS Trust supervision policy
- RCSLT guidance on dysphagia training, provided for institutions that run training courses.

Models of supervision

In our department we use several types of supervisory frameworks to ensure rigour in our practice. In relation to communication disorders, clinicians receive supervision related to both the clinical area and managerial issues. In relation to dysphagia, clinicians receive clinical supervision that is focused purely on this clinical area and does not cover management issues, such as human resources issues, signing of time sheets and holiday allocation. We will focus on dysphagia supervision throughout this chapter. In the UK SLTs are not trained to work in dysphagia when they graduate. Qualified SLTs have to undertake additional training to be able to work in dysphagia, and supervision is an important part of this training. Supervision for dysphagia in our department includes: individual supervision with a more experienced clinician, the development and implementation of a competency development plan to guide clinical skill development, and group supervision (four to six times annually). These are discussed further below.

Individual supervision

Individual dysphagia supervision starts when SLTs begin dysphagia work. Supervision takes place between the SLT and a more experienced therapist working in the clinical area. During the very first supervision meeting, the purpose is solely to design a competency development programme. This guides the SLT in the development of their skills in dysphagia. A mix of theoretical and practical activity is planned to support the SLTs to develop their skills, competence and confidence. Subsequent supervisions, which initially take place between weekly and monthly, will review and feedback on learning activities, and review cases that are being seen by the junior therapist and his/her supervising therapist. See Box 7.1 for an example competency plan set for the first two years for a new graduate.

Once the SLT has completed their competency plan, individual clinical supervision continues on a regular basis. Supervision meetings are usually every other month and take about an hour to an hour and a half. The format of the sessions includes a general discussion about how the SLT is feeling about the caseload and their skills and management. Individual cases are then discussed. The EBP 'triad' model is used to guide these discussions, (Sackett *et al.*, 1996). Assessment and management is reviewed and reflected upon. Future intervention is discussed in relation to what is known about the patient, the evidence base, and the supervisor and supervisee's clinical experience. Supervision notes are retained and referred to so over time both the supervisor and supervisee have a developing summary of clinical intervention and planning. Clinical discussions are noted in the patient notes when supervision has finished and supervision notes are retained for future reference. An example of an evidence-based case discussion is shown in Box 7.2.

In addition to supporting clinical decision-making regarding individual cases, the clinical supervision meetings help to prepare clinicians for multidisciplinary discussion about clients. In the clinical field of learning disabilities, many decisions are made in multidisciplinary 'best interests' meetings (Joyce, 2007). In these meetings intervention is considered for patients who have difficulties making their own decisions. They are attended by families, care staff and multidisciplinary professionals. The intervention options and their risks and benefits are considered. Preparing for multidisciplinary discussion in clinical supervision using an EBP framework is invaluable. It gives the SLTs confidence to take part or even lead these meetings.

Group supervision

Dysphagia group supervision takes place on a regular basis four to six times per year. All the qualified SLTs are required to attend, whether or not they have completed their dysphagia training. In addition we have some highly trained SLT assistants who undertake support work in dysphagia, and they also attend sessions. Group supervision sessions have a number of activities, outlined below.

- *Caseload monitoring.* All SLTs report on the size of their current dysphagia caseloads, including the proportion of patients who require a high level of activity (one to two contacts per week) or who are being monitoring (one contact every six weeks to three months). This allows us to discuss and monitor referral rates across the department, and to take an evidence-based approach to caseload management. There is a growing range of evidence that indicates the negative impact of large caseloads on clinicians (Blood *et al.*, 2002; Coffey and Coleman, 2001). It is also supported by experience within the department.

Box 7.1 Example competency plan

Throughout the development period:

- Small but gradually increasing caseload
- Directly supervised clinical work developing to individual management with regular discussion with dysphagia specialist
- Observation of other SLTs
- Regular supervision moving from every other week, to every other month
- Attendance at dysphagia peer supervision group, with increasingly active involvement, e.g. presenting a case, leading a critical appraisal
- Attendance at regional dysphagia Special Interest Group (SIG)
- Guided research

Months 1–6

- Complete work for the post basic dysphagia training course (attended recently)
- Research to be coursework focused
- Keep log of observations of other SLTs. This would include details about patients observed, assessments, intervention and challenges to case management
- Attend any available training for carers
- Read RCSLT and departmental standards and policies

Months 7–12

- Building good awareness of other multidisciplinary team members while working with small number of cases
- Attendance at external Learning Difficulties peer support groups
- Observation of SLTs in other clinical areas, e.g. adult neurology and paediatrics

Months 13–18

- Collaborative training for carer/staff with another SLT
- Develop videofluoroscopy experience, via observations with adult neurology dept
- Presentation of case at dysphagia peer supervision

Months 19–24

- Active member of peer supervision group
- Carrying out individual training
- Multidisciplinary working
- Research self directed – case based and interest led
- Beginning attendance at further training courses

Box 7.2 Example of an evidence-based case discussion undertaken in supervision

Marie is a 29-year-old woman with profound and multiple learning disabilities. She has lived all her life with her parents, and attends a day centre 5 days a week. Marie has never been reported to suffer from chest infections in the past. She has been referred to SLT because of increased coughing on all consistencies, longer mealtimes, mealtimes that appear distressing and deteriorating general health. Assessment was guided by the 'best available' evidence which were consensus documents. During assessment Marie coughed on all food and drink, and her breathing became rapid and noisy. Her mealtimes were long and difficult, she was very low weight, and had limited oral skills.

We reviewed Marie's history in supervision. There was no report of chest infections in Marie's history so we considered whether a videofluoroscopic swallow study would help us decide which intervention option(s) would be best for Marie.

Discussion was framed around the three components of EBP:

- *Patient preference*: Discussed Marie's distress at mealtimes, capacity for consent, and family and staff's opinions with regards to Marie's difficulty and SLT input;
- *Clinical experience*: Reflected on similar cases managed previously and success of videofluoroscopy on case management, suitability of patient for assessment;
- *Best available evidence*: Reflected on evidence indicating that videofluoroscopy is the 'gold standard' assessment (Langmore *et al.*, 1991; Mathers-Schmidt and Kurlinski, 2003; Stoeckli *et al.*, 2003; Tohara *et al.*, 2003), and that it would provide information required in this case.

On the basis of the discussion of Marie's case and consideration of the above, it was agreed that a videofluoroscopy would be recommended.

Therefore, where caseload size is becoming too demanding, work is reallocated to other SLTs.
- *Critical appraisal of papers.* Over the last decade, there has been an increasing awareness about the validity and robustness of the evidence we use to guide our clinical decision-making. As clinicians we need to be able to find appropriate and valid evidence to support our decision-making. Integral to this is the ability to judge the evidence, that is, critical appraisal (Hill and Spittlehouse, 2001). In order to develop and maintain our skills and confidence in critical appraisal we review and evaluate relevant research papers as a group. We then discuss the relevance and application of the findings for our patient group, and our particular clinical setting. Where relevant we decide on future actions as a team.
- *Presentation of cases.* In group supervision, we share clinical practice and learn from each other by presenting and reflecting on at least one clinical case at each meeting (Duffy, 2007; Johns, 1995; Todd and Freshwater, 1999). The

cases are usually ones that have challenged SLTs. Clinicians are also encouraged to present cases that they feel went well and to reflect on why. There are learning outcomes for both the presenting SLT and the rest of the group.

- *Videofluoroscopic swallow study (VFSS) review.* The VFSS is widely accepted to be the 'gold standard' assessment tool in dysphagia (Langmore *et al.*, 1991; Mathers-Schmidt and Kurlinski, 2003; Stoeckli *et al.*, 2003; Tohara *et al.*, 2003). There are concerns raised in the literature that SLTs do not always agree on what they see; that is, the inter-rater reliability is poor (Tohara *et al.*, 2003). There is evidence that the more videofluoroscopies SLTs observe, and the more they rate and discuss them together, the better inter-rater agreement becomes. We do not carry out many videofluoroscopies per year in our service. In order to maximize our skills, and reliability, every videofluoroscopy that is done in our department is brought to the next group supervision session to be presented and discussed.

- *Audit and research dissemination.* In order to learn from our own initiatives and build on developments within the department, audits or projects undertaken are presented to the group. They are then discussed and further action is decided upon. In this way we create and develop our own local evidence base. We also have some research-active practitioners. This forum allows them to present information locally for peer review before their work is opened to a wider audience. It also encourages the generation of new ideas for further research.

- *Discussion of continuing professional development.* As NHS resources are finite and access to external training is often limited, SLTs are required to provide evidence that they are engaging in CPD activity. When SLTs attend external training they share information with the rest of the team so that the other SLTs can update their knowledge and use this to inform their evidence-based case management.

An example of discussions held in group supervision is shown in Box 7.3.

Reflections on supervision

EBP is often felt to be challenging and it is frequently reported that clinicians do not have enough time to do it, due to many other demands. In our department, although a comparatively large amount of time is spent in clinical supervision, it is valued by all members of staff. Attendance is high, and this has continued for the eight years the system has been running. The group supervision is particularly successful in terms of allowing clinicians a non-judgemental and safe environment to review their strengths and needs, and to ask colleagues for support with difficult cases. It has been successful in maintaining skills in videofluoroscopy interpretation, and in developing skills in critical appraisal. Individual supervision has been invaluable in providing therapists with the opportunity to ask for support in activities they find particularly challenging, and has proved particularly important when SLTs are managing complex and difficult cases. In particular, SLTs report they find it very useful at times of patient death. It also allows seamless management of cases, where treating SLTs have to take time off and the supervising SLT can take over management. I hope that the examples described prove helpful in guiding other departments in their own supervision activities.

Box 7.3 Integrating new evidence into practice through discussion in group supervision sessions

The UK National Patient Safety Agency (NPSA) identified dysphagia as a key risk area for people with learning disabilities (NPSA, 2004). During discussion of this document at group supervision we became aware that our local Risk Management department were not necessarily aware of the patients we managed who were at chronic risk from dysphagia. We invited the risk manager to attend group supervision, and together we identified five areas for reporting to the risk department, informed by experience, the NPSA report and research conducted locally (Crawford *et al.*, 2007). These included:

- Chronic risk from dysphagia
- Non-compliance of carers
- Non-compliance of staff
- Choking
- Acute incident.

We have since started recording areas of risk through individual supervision, and registering this with the Risk Management department. The SLT department is evaluating the results, in order to identify the proportion of patients who present as being at high risk for dysphagia in our service. We will discuss the clinical implications of these findings at future meetings. Further investigation into appropriate intervention and management is planned.

References

Blood, G., Ridenour, J.S., Thomas, E.A., Qualls, C.D. and Hammer, C.S. (2002) Predicting job satisfaction among speech-language pathologists working in public schools. *Language, Speech and Hearing Services in Schools*, **33**, 282–290.

Coffey, M. and Coleman, M. (2001) The relationship between support and stress in forensic community mental health nursing. *Journal of Advanced Nursing*, **34** (3), 397–407.

Crawford, H., Leslie, P. and Drinnan, M.J. (2007) Compliance with dysphagia recommendations by carers of adults with intellectual impairment. *Dysphagia*, **22** (4), 326–334.

Duffy, A. (2007) A concept analysis of reflective practice: determining its value to nurses. *British Journal of Nursing*, **16** (22), 1400–1407.

Hill, A. and Spittlehouse, C. (2001) What is critical appraisal? Retrieved 13 October 2009 from http://www.medicine.ox.ac.uk/bandolier/painres/download/whatis/What_is_critical_appraisal.pdf

Johns, C. (1995) The value of reflective practice for nursing. *Journal of Clinical Nursing*, **4** (1), 23–30.

Joyce, T. (2007) *Best interests: Guidance on determining the best interests of adults who lack the capacity to make a decision (or decisions) for themselves (England and Wales).* London: British Psychological Society and Department of Health.

Langmore, S.E., Schatz, K. and Olson, N. (1991) Endoscopic and videofluoroscopic evaluations of swallowing and aspiration. *Annals of Otology, Rhinology and Laryngology,* **100**, 678–681.

Mathers-Schmidt, B.A. and Kurlinski, M. (2003) Dysphagia evaluation practices: Inconsistencies in clinical assessment and instrumental examination decision-making. *Dysphagia,* **18**, 114–125.

National Patient Safety Agency (2004) Understanding the patient safety issues for people with learning disabilities. Available from the NPSA web site, www.npsa.nhs.uk.

Sackett, D.L., Richardson, W.S., Rosenberg, W. and Haynes, R.B. (1997) *Evidence-Based Medicine: How to Practice and Teach EBM.* London: Churchill Livingstone.

Sackett, D.L., Rosenberg, W.M.C., Gray, J.A.M., Haynes, R.B. and Richardson, W.S. (1996) Evidence-based medicine: What it is and what it isn't. *British Medical Journal,* **312**, 71–72.

Stoeckli, S., Huisman, T., Seifert, B. and Martin-Harris, B. (2003) Interrater reliability of videofluoroscopic swallow evaluation. *Dysphagia,* **13** (1), 53–57.

The Royal College of Speech and Language Therapists (2006) *Communicating Quality* (3rd edn). London: RCSLT.

Todd, G. and Freshwater, D. (1999) Reflective practice and guided discovery: clinical supervision. *British Journal of Nursing,* **8** (20), 1383–1389.

Tohara, H., Saitoh, E., Mays, K., Kuhlemeier, and Palmer, J. (2003) Three tests for predicting aspiration without videofluoroscopy. *Dysphagia,* **18**, 126–134.

Meeting skill gaps and training needs (commentary on Section Two)

Hazel Roddam and Jemma Skeat

The chapters in this section have highlighted various ways that we can develop evidence-based practice (EBP) skills and knowledge as speech and language therapists (SLTs). An important question though is 'what are we aiming for?' That is, what constitutes the minimum skill set or competency level for SLTs in terms of EBP? Searching electronic databases and critical appraisal of published research literature continue to be the two predominant skills gaps that are identified by many SLTs. Muir-Gray (2001) recommends basic competence levels in searching and appraisal of research for all healthcare practitioners 'who make decisions about patients or groups of patients' (p. 330). These are not the only skills relevant to EBP, however. It is essential that we also have the skills to implement changes in our clinical practice and to measure the impact of those changes: these too are integral elements of the EBP cycle.

This brief discussion will touch on ways in which SLTs can access these basic skill sets. It will also consider what may constitute more advanced skills, including how essential they are, and how they might add further benefit for individuals or for services/teams.

Existing resources to build basic EBP skill sets

It is recognized that understanding how to access and appraise the research literature may be a specific challenge for practising SLTs who did not have this as a component of their initial qualification. The first two chapters in this section have illustrated ways in which these elements of EBP are now being incorporated into professional training courses, to ensure that our newly qualified practitioners are appropriately skilled and confident. There is a need for this formal training approach to be complemented by ongoing training and skill development in the clinical setting – not only for those clinicians who have not been exposed to this in their training years, but to continue to support and develop those who have had this exposure. Satty and Gina (Chapter 6) and Hannah (Chapter 7) illustrate two different approaches that generate opportunities within the workplace for SLTs to acquire new skills as well as to have refresher and update sessions.

There are many resources that can support the development of these skills whether within formal training or ongoing continuing professional development. There are a profusion of publications and guides on research appraisal, literature searching, and other skill areas available to buy. However, we would like to point out the wealth of resources that are freely available within the public domain. We would also like to highlight that the resources that should be considered do not only include those written by and for SLTs, particularly when it comes to generic skill areas such as searching literature databases or understanding research methodologies. The School of Health and Related Research (ScHARR) at the University of Sheffield, UK hosts a wide range of free access tutorials, including some excellent guides to searching electronic databases (http://www.shef.ac.uk/scharr/ir/netting/). The Critical Appraisal Skills Programme (CASP) at the University of Oxford, UK (http://www.phru.nhs.uk/Pages/PHD/CASP.htm) also has excellent critical appraisal checklists freely available on their web site, and many people find these to be helpful to use either for their own reading or to support journal clubs or other group appraisal approaches. There are distinct checklists for a wide range of research designs; including randomized controlled trials, economic evaluation studies, cohort studies, case–control studies, diagnostic tool development, and qualitative research designs. Other publications that incorporate well-written guides to support clinicians to address these EBP processes include Crombie (1996); NHS Executive (1999); Greenhalgh and Donald (2000); Muir-Gray (2001), and Greenhalgh (2006). Critical evaluation of research findings needs to be underpinned by an awareness of research designs and a grasp of the nature of research questions that can be answered by contrasting designs. Tricia Greenhalgh wrote a most valuable series of introductory guides in the *British Medical Journal* (also published in Greenhalgh, 2006), and in particular we highly recommend you to look at her papers on identifying research designs (Greenhalgh, 1997a), understanding systematic reviews (Greenhalgh, 1997b), basic statistical considerations (Greenhalgh, 1997c, d), and the differences between qualitative and quantitative methodologies (Greenhalgh and Taylor, 1997).

One of our aims in developing this book was to highlight the need to consider the implementation of change in clinical practice, and this requires its own skill set. Bury and Mead (1998) suggest that lack of understanding of change processes acts as a predominant barrier to facilitating EBP. There are several resources to support skills and knowledge in understanding and influencing change in clinical practice. Some excellent resources are provided by the Institute for Healthcare Improvement http://www.ihi.org/IHI/Topics/Improvement/, and the National Institute for Clinical Studies (NICs) (http://www.nhmrc.gov.au/nics/).

Developing skills and competencies through continuing professional development

Skills and competences for EBP may be regarded as an essential component of continuing professional development (CPD). CPD may target these as discrete skills, but there is also the opportunity for CPD focusing on clinical topics to be underpinned by an evidence-based approach that reinforces the development and use of these skills. We would like to propose that it is timely for us all to become more discerning and expect that any clinical CPD courses should be more explicitly evidence-based than ever before. This means that any claims about assessment and treatment, including new ideas and approaches, are supported by evidence, with sources of data explicitly cited. Training workshops, conference presentations and other CPD events should be subjected to as much critical appraisal as a journal article; we need to ask what evidence there is, how strong it is, and to consider this information alongside our own clinical knowledge and patient preferences when applying what we have learned from CPD events to our practice. We believe that the professional bodies have a role to play in ensuring that CPD events meet these criteria.

Advanced EBP skills

So, there is a need for all SLTs to feel confident in these fundamental skills of EBP, is there any need for more advanced skills? If so, what would those be; and how can they be used to the maximum benefit? As in any discipline, individuals will be motivated to follow their own interests and some will have developed relative strengths in certain areas, which might include conducting database searches, understanding or applying certain research designs, or confidence in undertaking and/or interpreting statistical analyses. We would affirm that the most important skill for us all to cultivate is that of networking: to know who are the experts locally and how you can access their help if it is needed. Find out about services available from local medical librarians, other professional colleagues with research experience, and make links with local university staff. Knowing who to ask may be the most valuable skill of all. For service managers who recognize that they have members in their teams who have particular areas of interest and expertise – including newly qualified therapists who have the benefit of very recent learning on these topics – we would recommend that these strengths should be optimized for the benefit of all the staff. It will be far more efficient and effective to engage these individuals to assist in co-ordinating the development of service-level evidence-based policies and resources.

Summary

The identification of relevant skills gaps and training needs is essential at a personal level as well as across teams. The contributed chapters in the following section give a range of insights into ways in which this has been achieved in SLT services. For those who do not currently work within teams in this way, we would recommend that there are still useful indications for all levels of planning and delivery of SLT services. It should also be recognized that skills are required for all stages of the EBP cycle, although this section of the book has focused predominantly on finding and appraising published research sources.

References

Bury, T. and Mead, J. (1998) *Evidence-based Healthcare: A Practical Guide for Therapists*. Oxford: Butterworth-Heinemann.

Crombie, I. (1996) *The Pocket Guide to Critical Appraisal: A Handbook for Health Care Professionals*. London: BMJ Publishing Group.

Greenhalgh, T. (1997a) How to read a paper: Getting your bearings (deciding what the paper is about). *British Medical Journal*, 315, 243–246.

Greenhalgh, T. (1997b) How to read a paper: papers that summarise other papers (systematic reviews and meta analyses). *British Medical Journal*, 315, 672–675.

Greenhalgh, T. (1997c) How to read a paper: Statistics for the non-statistician. I: Different types of data need different statistical tests. *British Medical Journal*, 315, 364–366.

Greenhalgh, T. (1997d) How to read a paper: Statistics for the non-statistician. II: 'Significant' relations and their pitfalls. *British Medical Journal*, 315, 422–425.

Greenhalgh, T. (2006) *How to Read a Paper: The Basics of Evidence-Based Medicine* (3rd edn). London: Wiley-Blackwell.

Greenhalgh, T. and Donald, A. (2000) *Evidence Based Health Care Workbook*. London: BMJ Publishing Group.

Greenhalgh, T. and Taylor, R. (1997) How to read a paper: papers that go beyond numbers (qualitative research). *British Medical Journal*, 315, 740–743.

Muir-Gray, J.A. (2001) *Evidence-based Healthcare: How to Make Health Policy and Management Decisions* (2nd edn). London: Churchill Livingstone.

NHS Executive (1999) *Evidence-Based Health Care: An Open Learning Resource for Health-Care Practitioners. Unit 3. Appraising and Interpreting Evidence*. Luton: Critical Appraisal Skills Programme and Health Care Libraries Unit.

Section Three

Creating a supportive context for EBP

The role of leadership in creating evidence-based services

Karen Davies

Standards Manager, Skills for Health; formerly Professional Manager for Speech and Language Therapy, Trafford Primary Care Trust, UK

This chapter considers the role of clinical leadership in developing culture and capacity in evidence-based practice (EBP). It will focus on the importance of leadership in instigating and guiding change in response to new evidence. I will draw on my experience as a professional manager for the adult and children's speech and language therapy (SLT) services in a Primary Care Trust in the UK. In this role I worked with a team of 35 therapists and assistants providing a range of services, from early parent programmes through to specialist intervention for people with long term communication difficulties. The service design and quality is firmly based on the core professional standards found in 'Communicating Quality' (Royal College of Speech and Language Therapists [RCSLT], 2006), whilst, at the same time, fulfilling the expectations of external stakeholders, who have commissioned a number of specialist services for specific client groups. Responding to the needs of these commissioners has provided a considerable impetus to find, and to use, relevant evidence to develop services, as well as demanding that we actively collate and interpret evidence from our own practice to demonstrate the benefits that speech and language therapy can provide for those with limited communication.

As I reflect on my own growing understanding of EBP, I can begin to identify a number of key factors that have challenged and influenced the implementation of a more systematic approach to building services based on best evidence. My own role as a clinical lead has developed in the context of an organization that is required to fulfil the standards of a clear clinical governance framework. This has challenged me to provide assurance for service users and the wider organization that clinical decision-making across the service is based on up-to-date knowledge drawn from research and professional consensus. Whilst the responsibility for basing practice on the best available evidence lies with each practitioner, the role of clinical leadership is essential in creating an environment that promotes this at an organizational level and supports the process of change that will follow on from this. Using evidence to inform service development depends on good leadership that 'empowers team work, creates an open and questioning culture and ensures both the ethos and the day to day delivery of clinical governance remain an integral part of every service' (Halligan and Donaldson, 2001, p. 1414).

As a clinical lead, I have the responsibility for demonstrating the benefits of new service developments for patients. This has created the opportunity to evaluate practice and to introduce a structured process for using evidence from research, together with collating and interpreting evidence from our own local practice. This has been dependent on enabling practitioners to develop skills in using evidence to improve practice.

The following sections incorporate examples of how we have used evidence to lead change across our SLT service. I have focused on a range of initiatives that have been developed internally, within the service, as well as externally, through participation in wider organizational approaches. I have found it valuable to reflect on the literature around influencing workplace culture and supporting staff to work in new ways and hope that this overview will be helpful to others who are leading SLT services.

Communicating the vision

Leaders of clinical services need to recognize the extent to which they influence the perception of EBP by staff. In my role, I have aimed to develop an approach that avoids considering EBP as an isolated element, disconnected from the way services are designed and delivered. We can often feel defeated by a belief that it is difficult to relate evidence to our interventions because of limited research and complex and demanding work contexts. This can inhibit interest in using evidence to inform practice and reduce enthusiasm to apply research to our routine decision making. I have aimed to create an environment where it has become expected that practitioners will seek out the available evidence before commencing on a specific treatment or new initiative, and where time is given to evaluating the impact of these local changes, in order to generate further substantive evidence.

A recent example in the UK has been the role for SLTs in the Sure Start programme, which has focused on language promotion through working collaboratively with early years workers and parents. Innovative programmes were set up in response to a national initiative and local needs. They were then evaluated and shared with other SLT services through professional networks. In this situation, the available evidence was not in the form of a comprehensive research study with clear conclusions, but required therapists to examine the evidence for different interventions and integrate that with what was known of their own local context. Over time, many of these initiatives have been evaluated and evidence is gradually emerging to indicate which have been the most successful programs (de Jager and Houston, 2006; Sawyer *et al.*, 2007). Leaders of clinical services needed to convey a vision that demonstrated the value of creating, as well as collating, best evidence in order to deliver effective local services.

Learning from the evidence

The organizational approach to learning can facilitate or hinder the implementation of best practice. When learning is restricted it becomes impossible to implement new and emerging evidence of best practice. Senge (1994) defined a 'learning organisation' as one that places learning as a core element of its functioning. This capacity to utilize learning is central to supporting organizational development:

> learning is something achieved by individuals, but 'learning organisations' can configure themselves to maximise, mobilise and retain this learning potential (Davies and Nutley, 2000, p. 998).

Whilst gaining new knowledge about best practice depends on the learning of individuals, it is the organization that supports the translation of this knowledge into improved services. A learning organization must go beyond supporting practitioners to increase their knowledge and skills in a specific area, and aim to develop deeper understanding with outcomes that are more extensive and radical for the organization. Learning organizations are constantly striving to improve their services, and are therefore routinely seeking out new evidence which can then inform innovation and change.

As a clinical lead, I have attempted to promote a learning organization in our service through ensuring that learning is at the centre of decision making. Learning is achieved through challenging practice, recognizing ineffective intervention and actively seeking evidence to inform service planning. Creating the environment that encourages learning requires leadership to utilize regular meetings which support the operational running of services. Our team meetings, supervision meetings and planning meetings include a standing item that allows team members to contribute critiques of articles, resources and initiatives, with specific questions about how this contributes to the evidence we already have and how it should influence our practice. This is what Nutley *et al.* (2000) describe as leadership that aims to 'transform practice styles so that the use of best evidence is an ongoing routine activity' (p. 5).

SLT leaders must also ensure that the profession contributes to the wider organization, 'sharing knowledge throughout the organisation is one key to developing learning capacity' (Davies and Nutley, 2000, p. 1001). SLTs are often in unique roles that span across organizations, such as health, education and social services, and are therefore in a valuable position to share learning from their experiences of using best evidence. We have found that setting up a network with a range of different professionals provides an excellent forum for championing learning from research in order to improve services for patients and users. Other examples of how this could be achieved include a Clinical Effectiveness Network or a Research and Development Group that meets periodically to create the strategy for the service, review progress and support the practical implementation of EBP. This enables therapists to create a strategy that is directly relevant to their own service whilst also contributing to the wider organizational requirements. The function of the network is to provide the environment for dissemination of research, sharing best practice, plus encouraging research awareness amongst network members. Each member takes responsibility for championing EBP in their own work area and supports the implementation of clinically effective practice within their team. Networks can be created within a professional group or across a number of different professions but evidence is emerging of the real benefit of enabling learning across an organization rather than within isolated professional groups.

Creating a learning organization is not easy, particularly when practitioners have established ways of working and struggle with too little time to think differently.

There are tensions, too, when national direction focuses on achieving specific targets (such as reducing waiting times) that may discourage meaningful changes to services. At the present time, SLT services in the UK are preparing themselves for the challenges of independent commissioning of services by any agency, including non-statutory organizations. The possibility that practitioners will be required to provide intervention that is not evidence-based will require skilled leadership in influencing the commissioning process. Strong leadership, and an established culture of learning, will be essential in managing these tensions.

Supporting therapists to reflect on practice and review their services

As noted above, the clinical lead often sets the culture for SLT departments in relation to EBP. As such, it is essential that they have high expectations that standards of practice are grounded in best evidence, placing clinical effectiveness as the essential building block for practice. I have approached this through constantly re-emphasizing the need to focus on the evidence, together with using a range of practical tools to support service evaluation and review. EBP has to be a process that is integrated into the delivery of services rather than managed as a separate entity with a life of its own that then needs to be applied to practice.

Service planning, with all SLTs in the department involved, can be a real catalyst for evidence-focused service improvement. In our experience, this has prompted many practical opportunities to implement best evidence. As a result of these planning activities, we have developed a considerable number of evidence-based local policies, standards and guidelines. Standards can then be audited and services evaluated, allowing local teams to contribute to the evidence base. However, I would suggest that in order to most effectively enable therapists, the following points are essential first steps in this planning process:

- Acknowledge that opinion-based practice may be both inefficient and ineffective, and that there may be better ways of working that meet the needs of clients. Process mapping and designing care pathways are both very effective in identifying inefficient practices and processes (see the NHS Institute for Innovation and Improvement, www.institute.nhs.uk)
- Take time away from service delivery to evaluate current practice and plan developments: 'health services need to plan to develop the quality of their services' (Halligan and Donaldson, 2001, p. 1414).
- Incorporate time into weekly practice through timetabling a development session when jobs are restructured. This demonstrates the importance that the clinical lead places on ensuring services are designed according to up-to-date evidence.

Our experience has shown that therapists tend to be reluctant planners at a wider, whole service level, often becoming daunted by the need to record the steps required to improve services. Equally, leaders of services can be poor at engaging practitioners in the process of planning. Our teams are often animated as they

Table 9.1 Example of service planning proforma

Name:
Department:
Telephone Contact:
Date of Proposal:

Development Proposal Outline:

Identifying best practice:
  Where is the evidence for this approach?
  How practical is it within our context?
  How are other services involved?

Objectives:

Methods:

Anticipated benefits to patients:

Costs:
  Time
  Resources

Review Date:

Outcomes:
  How will they be recorded?
  How will they be shared with the team?
  If successful, how can the initiative be extended?

Follow up action:

discuss options for service improvement, but have difficulty maintaining progress and monitoring improvement. The clinical lead is essential in supporting momentum. We found that a highly effective way of ensuring that the impetus is maintained was achieved through using service development tools. Even the simplest planning tool that is incorporated into every opportunity to improve services can provide assurance that plans are carefully considered and informed by evidence. It also provides an excellent means of tracking progress throughout a development so that practitioners can recognize progress and identify points where progress has stagnated. Table 9.1 is an example of a proforma that is simple enough to prompt therapists to be concise and considered in planning service developments and to provide a record that monitors progress.

Enabling therapists to contribute to the evidence

Whilst practitioners are instrumental in ensuring evidence from research is applied to specific client groups, they are also at the forefront of generating the questions that need to be researched. In order to support practitioners to contribute to the evidence as well implement best practice, the clinical lead needs to create challenging opportunities that include:

- Supporting staff to undertake further study. This will challenge existing practice and improve a practitioner's reasoning. Professional development that focuses on improving a practitioner's understanding of research methods will lead to a more focused approach to service delivery.
- Actively developing partnerships with universities to enable practitioners to participate in teaching and research. This was specifically identified in a recent Government paper on Clinical Effectiveness in the UK, which stated 'we believe the health service can do more to harness more effectively the capacity of higher education to assist with delivering advances in medical practice' (Tooke, 2007, p. 6).
- Setting up interactive workshops to promote learning linked with the opportunity to plan service delivery. This has been identified as one of the most effective ways to change practice (O'Brien *et al.*, 2001). The timing and design of workshops is crucial to ensure that practitioners are engaged. I introduced a series of monthly lunch-time service improvement events, which were particularly successful in supporting practitioners through the stages of reviewing services and planning improvements. The combination of training in seeking out the evidence, practical planning around a specific project plus peer support enabled significant changes to take place across our service.
- Creating Clinical Effectiveness Champions who will support peers to undertake audit, evaluations and research. Nominating representatives from each area of a service to support their colleagues in developing and maintaining effective practice generates genuine participation from every team member. The role of the clinical lead in this situation is setting the direction of the work of the champions and supporting the practical processes of ensuring a working group achieves clear goals.

Reflections on sustaining change

An essential skill for helping me to balance my priorities and resolve some of the tensions that inevitably arise in trying to embed EBP in service delivery has been the process of reflection. The questions shown in Box 9.1 have provided an excellent benchmark for measuring my own effectiveness as a clinical lead in promoting EBP across my own service.

Changes in working practices can only be sustained if they become established as the habits of a team or service. However, once new practices have been adopted, it can be easy to lose the impetus to remain rigorous in improving standards. There is a need to constantly re-energize and re-engage staff to support an ongoing commitment to reviewing the evidence for services. Nutley *et al.* (2000) comment that 'There is little doubt that making a reality of EBP will require careful analysis, skilful advocacy and great stamina' (p. 6). The task of enabling services to be grounded in the best evidence will be a continual process and service leaders will have to find continual reserves of energy to maintain the progress that users of our services should expect.

Box 9.1   Reflecting on the impact of leadership

- How am I involved in shaping strategy that supports EBP?
- How am I changing the culture of my work environment to encourage learning and consistent use of best evidence?
- How am I enabling my peers to value, use and contribute to EBP?
- How am I planning service delivery based on best evidence?
- In what ways have services improved for the user as a result of implementing best evidence?

References

Davies, H.T.O. and Nutley, S.M. (2000) Developing learning organisations n the new NHS. *British Medical Journal*, **320**, 998–1001.

de Jager, M. and Houston, A. (2006) Mainstreaming Sure Start speech and language therapy services. *Community Practitioner*, **79** (3), 80–83.

Halligan, A. and Donaldson, L. (2001). Implementing clinical governance: turning vision into reality. *British Medical Journal*, **322**, 1413–1417.

Nutley, S., Davies, H.T.O. and Tilley, N. (2000) Editorial: Getting research into practice. *Public Money & Management*, **20** (4), 3–6.

O'Brien, M.A., Freemantle, N., Oxman, A.D., Davis, D.A. and Herrin, J. (2001) Continuing education meetings and workshops: effects on professional practice and health care outcomes. *Cochrane Database of Systematic Reviews*, **1** (Article No. CD003030).

Royal College of Speech and Language Therapists (2006) *Communicating Quality* (3rd edn). London: RCSLT.

Sawyer, V., Pickstone, C. and Hall, D. (2007) *Promoting Speech and Language – a Themed Study in 15 Sure Start Local Programmes*. London: Department of Children, Families and Schools.

Senge, P.M. (1994) *The Fifth Discipline: the Art and Practice of the Learning Organization*. New York: Doubleday.

Tooke, J. (2007) *Report of the High Level Group on Clinical Effectiveness*. London: Department of Health.

10

Supporting staff to balance caseload demands

Sean Pert

Principal Speech and Language Therapist, Community Clinic,
NHS Heywood, Middleton and Rochdale Community Healthcare, UK

A therapist's time and how this is allocated is frequently cited as a significant obstacle to the implementation of evidence-based practice (EBP). When therapists have heavy caseload demands, they may have little time to reflect on their practice. Newly qualified therapists may be particularly overwhelmed by the responsibility of a long waiting list, at a time when they are just developing their skills. Management of long waiting lists is often simplistic, with rationing of time allocated per child, resulting in children being discharged, regardless of outcome. In this situation, with limited time for EBP, therapists are often left with no choice but to prioritize client contact above EBP and reflective practice.

This chapter describes a typical service in England, delivered in 11 community clinics in a specific primary care trust in the north-west of England. Community clinics are National Health Service (NHS) buildings where health services are delivered to the local community. A Trust is the local organization which commissions non-acute health services on behalf of the NHS. The community clinic model has been long established in the UK, usually consisting of a lone therapist providing one-to-one assessment and treatment to children referred in the local area. Newly qualified therapists frequently have at least one day of community clinic work as part of their timetable. In areas with large geographical areas to cover, and/or with limited or no speech and language therapy (SLT) coverage by the Local Education Department for nursery and school settings, the community clinic model continues to provide a much demanded service. Some areas have abandoned the traditional direct service delivery model in favour of indirect therapy models (for example, training programmes for parents and classroom staff), recognizing that even rationing therapy sessions cannot meet the demands placed upon the service.

Our community clinic service has an open referral system. In common with other NHS services, the service is free. The team provides assessment, diagnosis and therapy packages for children aged 0–18 years, although the majority of clients are aged three to seven years. Most clients live within a 10-minute walk of their local clinic. The service receives between four to five hundred referrals per annum.

These referrals are mainly clients new to the service but may also include clients who have been previously discharged and re-referred. On first contact, clients may have undiagnosed difficulties such as autistic spectrum disorder or learning difficulties. The community clinic team identify such clients and refer them to specialist therapists and services. The service is delivered by 4.9 whole time equivalent (WTE) speech-language pathologists (or SLTs) all of whom work full or part-time for the service. 1.65 WTE SLT assistants provide outreach care in schools.

Over time, the service faced steadily increasing referral rates (approximately 10–12% each year) and each team member was faced with long waiting lists. Although screening appointments were offered within eight weeks of referral (a target for the NHS Trust governing the service), further assessment and, where appropriate, therapy provision were not provided until 13–24 months after referral. These huge waiting times produced an enormous strain on staff in terms of low morale, a high volume of telephone and written complaints (on average 14 complaints per month) and a feeling of isolation, as staff worked alone at the clinics to provide a service.

The challenges of implementing EBP in a busy service

In this context, providing an evidence-based service presented several challenges. The demand for therapist's time and attention to be focused on assessment and intervention meant that time for reflection and review of one's own practice was limited. Similarly, therapists found it difficult to have time for searching and identifying evidence relevant to their practice.

Team discussions identified that therapists had different clinical practices that varied according to training and experience. Most therapists had not changed their practice since qualifying and there was no consistent use of a standard approach to therapy across the service. A variety of methods were employed with no reflection on how effective they were and no attempts to link therapy to current research findings. For example, all therapists had received training in the Derbyshire Language Scheme, 'an intervention programme which targets early language skills' (Masidlover, 2004). However, none routinely used the assessment materials or detailed therapy manuals, despite these being readily available. Instead, therapists used tasks adapted from the scheme. This made evaluation of the effectiveness of the programme impossible. Similarly, therapists reported that they used the Metaphon approach (Dean et al., 1990) but had not referred to the original materials since completing their training and did not use the assessment and therapy materials.

Some team members, already under pressure to reduce waiting times, reported that they had no time to review their therapeutic techniques and wished to adapt their knowledge into an eclectic therapy package. However, less experienced team members found it difficult to know how to deliver therapy packages and write appropriate therapy goals. SLT assistants (SLTAs) were confused by the varying approaches often presented as the same therapy package by different therapists.

Several therapists reported that they did not have easy access to normative data. This led to additional waiting list pressures, as children were placed on waiting lists for therapy if there was any doubt that they had 'age-appropriate' skills. A typical example was phonological processes. Therapists referred to old normative data and were unaware of recent research.

In addition to time pressures, there was a level of discomfort with the idea of reflective practice. SLTs were not comfortable discussing cases and caseload management as this had been their sole responsibility. For a few therapists, change of any sort was extremely threatening, and some felt that the team leader had no authority to change the therapeutic practices of the team members. There were also knowledge barriers, as team members unfamiliar with literature searches and evaluating research papers often failed to differentiate between different levels of evidence when attempting to apply evidence to practice. For example, a team member might read and value a non-peer reviewed article above one from a peer-reviewed journal. Awareness of professional guidelines was high, as members of the UK professional body, the Royal College of Speech and Language Therapists are sent a copy and they are available online (RCSLT, 2006). However, few therapists had actually referred to the guidelines.

An approach was needed that would reduce time pressures on therapists and lead to better caseload management. This would support therapists to have more time for reflective practice. We strongly felt that this approach should not just be about rationing the hours available to children, but should be evidence-driven. At the same time, we identified a need to positively encourage staff to become open, reflective practitioners, and to have the skills necessary to evaluate and apply evidence to practice.

Reflecting on the evidence

Therapists were given the opportunity to reflect on their current practices, and to compare this to the evidence. The RCSLT guidelines (2006) acted as a framework for these team discussions. Many therapists, having observed a 6-week episode of care during training, assumed that this common practice was best practice. There is now strong evidence to support longer episodes of care. Law et al. (2003) found that '... interventions lasting longer than eight weeks may be more effective than those lasting less than eight weeks' (p. 15). Discussion of how normative data are collected and analysed challenged the belief held by some team members that normative data were 'hard facts' and increased their awareness of how to evaluate and apply research data to real clients. It also became clear that therapists assumed that individual therapy was more effective than group therapy. As with many areas of clinical practice, the answer may depend on several factors (such as the presenting disorder and frequency of therapy input). However, there is emerging evidence that group therapy is as effective as individual therapy. Boyle et al. (2007) found '... no significant differences ... between individual and group modes' (p. 89) for children aged 6–11 years receiving language therapy. Previously, SLTAs had a restricted role in therapy, usually carrying out the final therapy sessions for a child in the school environment. Since recent research indicated that SLTAs were as effective as therapists in delivering therapy (Boyle et al. 2007) we considered that better use of our SLTA time was indicated. The RCSLT guidelines further indicated that 'Parents ... should receive appropriate support and guidance to enable them to play a full and appropriate part in supporting their child …' (RCSLT, 2006, p. 243). Thus, the involvement of parents in the service would be an important element to an evidence-based service.

Meeting the challenges: an evidence-based service

One of the changes introduced was a group therapy option. Each clinic offered small group therapy (between two and eight children). Two 'first treatment' groups were run in each clinic, one for children with speech disorders (articulation difficulties, phonological delay and phonological disorder) and language disorders (language delay and language disorder). Other specific groups were then offered according to the clinical needs of the caseload (for example, an 's-cluster group' for children who reduced s-cluster production to a single consonant). SLTA time was reallocated to allow more work alongside therapists.

A unique model of group therapy was developed, in order to meet the need for flexibility in service provision. Specifically our 'first treatment' groups do not vary from week to week (i.e. there is no sequence of skills, with those taught on week one an essential prerequisite for week two). They are designed to teach the basic skills and also those skills required to access individual therapy if needed subsequently. Flexibility is ensured as children may leave the group if they achieve their aims and new children may join at any stage, instead of waiting for a new group to commence several weeks into the future.

As part of our redesign of the service to support greater capacity and reduce waiting lists, it was important that the service also allow greater parent involvement. Parent information sessions were built into the group therapy package. The sessions included information about typical development of language skills or speech skills in children. An explanation of the therapy activities and how parents could practise these skills at home was given. At the end of group sessions, therapists produced written and verbal feedback that helped to develop group activities to suit the needs of the families. We also found that less experienced team members could benefit from being supported in delivering pre-written information to parents, and so developed their presentation and interaction skills.

Therapist involvement in the service redesign

As noted above, some SLTs in the service were wary of reflective practice and change. It was important to engage therapists in the process of change, in order to allow ownership and to support implementation of the new service model. It was also critical to support the development of strong skills in the identification, review and application of the evidence.

SLTs required reassurance that EBP was a priority for the team and central to service redevelopment. The team leader set up peer support groups, and divided standard team meetings into two clear segments: an information sharing and planning segment, followed by a continuing professional development (CPD) segment. Clear targets were developed for each therapist, linked to these CPD segments. These targets would include a skill required to identify and embed

EBP. For example, one team member may have a personal target of developing literature search skills while another might focus on reviewing and evaluation skills. These staff would then support their peers to use the identified evidence and facilitate discussions on how this evidence could be used to develop clinical practice. These sessions were reinforced by asking staff to document their reflections on actual case discussions and relate their clinical decisions to clinical guidelines, care pathways and the evidence base. This approach was similar to the problem-based (case based) learning approach now used by several universities. We used case discussion as a learning technique in order to demonstrate to therapists that EBP is central to client care. Case discussions made EBP real for therapists. After several months therapists began to appreciate that there may be several answers to a question, and that many questions in speech and language therapy have yet to be answered. Therapists have now experienced carrying out literature searches, reviewing clinical guidelines and accessing specialist advisors, driven by the needs of a particular client. This drive is important as it constantly reminds the team that EBP is a tool for improving client care, and not an academic exercise.

In order to move ahead with redesigning the service around the evidence, the team decided to produce a client care pathway and devise a therapy manual, based on group therapy options proposed by the team leader. In this way, what was initially perceived to be an arbitrary management decision could be 'owned' by the team, as they would decide the form of the therapy provision and how to monitor it. Team members with EBP experience were asked to lead the development of this manual. Team meetings held over 12 months were used to examine progress and set targets in the creation of the care pathway and therapy manuals. During this time, team members were encouraged to try out techniques and discuss them at the team meeting.

In order to further support EBP in the service, particularly with regard to allocation of children to the waiting list, up-to-date normative data were identified through a series of literature searches carried out by team members. Therapists were asked to disseminate their findings at team meetings. Those therapists who were able to carry out literature searches facilitated other team members. This peer-to-peer learning and support was crucial in establishing EBP as a valid and time-effective activity. Therapists saw that by referring to the latest research they were able to provide parents with the latest information and have confidence in diagnosing presenting disorders. In particular, those children within normal limits could be discharged with appropriate advice rather than waiting to achieve adult-like speech and language patterns.

Evaluation of an evidence-based service redesign

The service was transformed by the service redesign and the changes have been supported by staff who previously questioned the benefits or use of EBP. Access to the service has improved dramatically as the 'first treatment' groups provide the initial episode of care within one week to four months of referral (down from 24 months). No community clinic has a waiting time for therapy over four months. The number of children waiting for therapy declined month-on-month from over

250 to around 20–30 children for the whole service. Complaints dropped dramatically over a year until no more waiting time complaints were received. In fact, feedback from parents was overwhelmingly positive. Parents reported that they felt more confident about supporting their child. Parents also mentioned that an opportunity to meet other parents of children with speech and language difficulties was highly valued.

The team continue to develop their EBP skills, and crucially, to apply them in case discussions and in improving both individual and group therapy. The team won the Trust award for outstanding service and has a more positive attitude to the community clinic caseload.

However, this approach has not been without its challenges. For example, reallocating SLTA time was initially extremely unpopular with the SLTAs themselves. They feared that therapists would not appreciate their skill level, and would use their time for mundane administrative tasks. Support from the team leader to ensure that therapy tasks and administrative tasks were shared between the therapist and SLTA was required.

For other staff who initially needed some additional encouragement to see that the service redesign could have positive impacts for the service, as well as for individual clients, we encouraged them to actively assist us with a service review after six months.

Reflections

For many services in the NHS in England, there is a danger that service redesign and change may be imposed as a reaction to service-user complaints and underfunding is often blamed for long waiting times. However, ensuring that the available staffing is used effectively is more productive than simply demanding more staff when there is often little chance of further funds being released. Another common strategy has been the rationing of therapy, with the aim of ensuring the continuation of a service with realistic waiting times. EBP helps the profession to challenge this short sighted view of client care.

We recognized that our therapists had a genuine commitment to providing ongoing continuity of care, which was potentially in conflict with the service targets for ensuring efficient case management. Our experience has shown that rather than being a luxury, examining the client pathway and ensuring that therapy is effective in meeting the clients' needs, ensures a smooth running system. Rationing therapy merely pays lip service to client needs whereas the delivery of focused evidence based care means that the client will require fewer or no further episodes. Using the evidence to guide us, we were able to balance our caseloads, which has led to more balanced SLTs, who can devote time to both clinical care, and reflective practice.

The introduction of a requirement for EBP and the keeping of a reflective record of continuing professional development has been a major driver in the UK. Active support from team leaders and managers to develop their skills in the context of real-life clients and work situations will empower SLTs to deliver the best possible care, and will also ensure real service benefits and efficiency.

References

Boyle, J., McCartney, E., Forbes, J. and O'Hare, A. (2007) A randomised controlled trial and economic evaluation of direct versus indirect and individual versus group modes of speech and language therapy for children with primary language impairment. *Health Technology Assessment*, **11** (25), 11–60.

Dean, E., Howell, J. and Walters, D. (1990) *Metaphon Resource Pack*. Windsor, UK: NFER-Nelson.

Law, J., Garrett, Z. and Nye, C. (2003) Speech and language therapy interventions for children with primary speech and language delay or disorder (Review). *The Cochrane Database of Systematic Reviews*, **3** (Art. No.: CD004110).

Masidlover, M. (2004) Derbyshire Language Scheme- Programme details. Retrieved 7 October 2009 from http://www.derbyshire-language-scheme.co.uk/Programme.htm

Royal College of Speech and Language Therapists (2006) *Communicating Quality* (3rd edn). London: RCSLT.

11

A model of clinician-researcher collaboration in a community setting

Conducting and evaluating clinical research in a multidisciplinary community based paediatric rehabilitation setting

Parimala Raghavendra

Manager, Research and Innovation, Division of Research and Innovation, Novita Children's Services, South Australia

This chapter discusses a model of involving clinicians in producing and evaluating the research evidence; a clinician–researcher collaboration that was utilized in a community-based paediatric rehabilitation setting with specific examples from speech and language therapy (SLT). Novita Children's Services, South Australia (Novita, formerly known as Crippled Children's Association of SA Inc., established in 1939) is a non-government, community-based organization that provides services to children with physical disabilities. Novita's services include therapy, equipment and family support, and we assist over 1300 children with physical and severe multiple disabilities or acquired brain injury and their families annually. Children assisted by Novita have cerebral palsy (approximately 65%), muscular dystrophy, spina bifida, Rett syndrome, or other conditions that result in a permanent physical disability. Novita employs family service co-ordinators, occupational therapists, orthotists, physiotherapists, psychologists, rehabilitation engineers and SLTs, totalling around 150 staff. Typically services are delivered in clients' homes, kindergartens and schools, or in community settings by multidisciplinary teams of therapists from five office sites in the Adelaide metropolitan area. Staff also visit one or more rural/country areas to support families and local service providers.

Bridging the research–practice gap

Novita, like other health care organizations, has had difficulty bridging the 'research to practice gap'. Research has traditionally been conducted within university and teaching hospital settings by academic faculty and/or researchers rather than in community organizations like Novita. Further, research outcomes are published in peer-reviewed journals or textbooks, or presented at conferences, and listening to and/or reading these findings does not readily translate to implementing or using it in our practice. Alongside this gap, however, there is the greater emphasis and expectation of funding bodies on finding methods and strategies to facilitate the uptake of research outcomes into practice, policy development, and in developing and manufacturing new technologies that will benefit the public (Baxter, 2008; Blackstone, 2007). The field of knowledge translation (KT) is gaining recognition and momentum in medicine, allied health and other fields. Blackstone (2007) defines KT as, '... an umbrella term ... referring to a range of activities and processes designed to ensure the utilization of research-based knowledge' (p. 2). KT is closely linked to evidence-based practice (EBP). Involving end users of research in the entire research process has been advocated as a method to advance EBP and KT (Baxter, 2008; King *et al.*, 2008). King *et al.* (2008) have argued that for research to be relevant and valued, and research outcomes to have impact on practice and policy, research must be conducted by teams of practitioners, managers, researchers and clients/families.

Novita has had a history of senior management conducting and/or supporting research, and this approach was further strengthened by the creation of a Research and Development Department in 1996 within the Regency Park Rehabilitation Engineering division of Novita, now called NovitaTech, and by the establishment of the Clinical Research Department (CRD) in 1999. Both were initiatives of senior executives at Novita. The aims of the CRD were to conduct research into the most effective and efficient clinical assessments and interventions for clients of Novita and their families, facilitate a spirit of enquiry amongst clinicians within Novita, and to reduce the research–practice gap.

The clinician–research collaboration model at Novita

Coming from a SLT background and with formal research qualifications and experience, I was appointed to the clinical research manager role to develop a cohesive research program in therapy and clinical services. My role was to:

- develop a strategic research direction and a multidisciplinary research programme across allied health and paediatric rehabilitation;
- facilitate and co-ordinate staff to initiate research around priorities established by various disciplines;
- disseminate through publications and presentations; and
- develop joint research projects with university training schools.

Senior executives at Novita quickly realized that for research to be undertaken and outcomes to be utilized meaningfully, there needed to be involvement of clinicians in the entire research process. With support from the clinical managers of allied health, a senior SLT, a physiotherapist, and an occupational therapist were employed to work as research senior therapists for one and a half days per week and they started with varying levels of research knowledge and experience. In their remaining employment hours they provided clinical services to clients. Thus, the model of clinician–researcher collaboration was born at Novita. The research seniors formed the key link between clinicians and the CRD by encouraging clinicians to ask the critical questions, supporting staff to undertake research and also by conducting discipline based projects, disseminating research outcomes and promoting EBP activities within Novita. In 2001, a Director of Therapy Services was appointed with oversight for clinical research and all allied health staff, which helped to further develop a cohesive research programme. The programme was later expanded to include a research senior psychologist and family service co-ordinator. Both the CRD and the introduction of the model of clinician–researcher collaboration aimed to produce research evidence to support clinical management and decision making at Novita, and to facilitate clinicians at Novita to critically appraise and apply research evidence in practice.

Producing the research evidence

The CRD managed research ideas and projects in a number of ways.

- Clinician-initiated ideas. Often, these staff would be involved in doing the research with education and support from the CRD, with time provided for release from clinical duties. This happened substantially in the early days of the CRD.
- Project ideas were initiated and developed by senior therapists and managers of disciplines and then the project was undertaken by the research senior therapist of that profession.
- Project ideas were proposed to or initiated by allied health university programmes and selected by undergraduate honours students and these projects were co-supervised by university faculty and Novita staff.
- Ideas were developed and projects conducted jointly with researchers from hospitals and academic institutions based in Adelaide.

All research ideas were evaluated by a Clinical Research Subcommittee consisting of Novita staff and a parent of a Novita client. Projects needed to align with organizational and CRD's strategic directions of (1) enhancing participation of children and families in the community, (2) investigations of life span issues of clients and families and/or (3) evaluations of interventions and service delivery. Projects also needed to deliver meaningful outcomes for clients, families and staff. A total of 112 ideas have been approved over the nine years that the initiative has run to date; that is, around one project idea a month! Figure 11.1 shows the types of projects undertaken since the CRD was developed. Projects have included those where research questions are posed and projects conducted by Novita staff (Novita projects), student projects (honours and postgraduate), and joint projects with universities, which have either been collaborative (with researchers from Novita working alongside University staff) or externally managed, with Novita providing access to clients or data for university projects. Seventy-eight percent of ideas approved were from Novita clinicians and/or managers in therapy services and NovitaTech staff. The substantial number of projects initiated by Novita staff highlights the spirit of inquiry amongst staff and the drive to find research evidence for important clinical questions. Details of these projects are on the Novita web

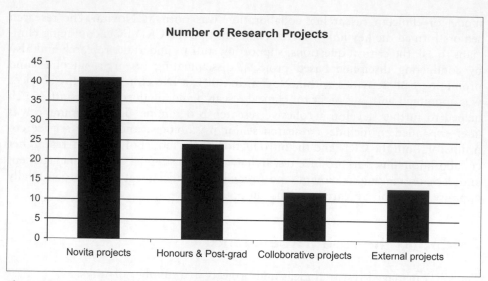

Figure 11.1   Number of research projects managed by the CRD at Novita.

site www.novita.org.au. Altogether, research and therapy staff have attracted a significant amount of external grant monies to support these high quality projects.

Producing the research evidence in SLT at Novita

SLTs were one of the most frequent groups to propose new ideas for research. The clinical questions posed by SLTs were often in the area of augmentative and alternative communication and paediatric dysphagia. One of the earliest questions posed by an individual clinician was, 'Can typically developing preschool children learn the meaning of graphic symbols through play?' (Manson *et al.*, 2000). The question arose out of the need to find the most effective and efficient methods to prepare typically developing peers to interact with classmates who use augmentative and alternative communication (AAC). The project found that children without disabilities learnt to recognize graphic symbols through playing with a speech generating device. Early projects such as this demonstrated the feasibility of a clinician–researcher model.

Two project ideas put forward by Novita SLTs and the clinical research manager were selected and completed as honours projects. One examined the school vocabulary use of 6-year-old typically developing children (Grace, 2004) and the other described the participation patterns of adolescents with and without physical disabilities and complex communication needs (McGregor, 2007). These projects have provided clinicians with information to use in practice (e.g. a vocabulary list for AAC systems) and generated knowledge around participation restrictions of young adults with disabilities.

Projects completed to date have been disseminated in a number of ways: presentations at state, national and international conferences, peer reviewed publications, and book chapters. The experiences of Novita SLTs with EBP have been published in the American-Speech–Language–Hearing Association newsletter (Olsson, 2003).

Supporting clinicians to evaluate and implement the evidence

In July 2000 the clinical research manager and key staff attended a three-day course on EBP conducted by the School of Physiotherapy, University of South Australia. Over the subsequent six years, using a Train-the-Trainer model, most managers and therapists were trained in EBP. The CRD found that the hierarchy of evidence model used in evidence-based medicine, and the tools used to evaluate research, were not suitable to appraise research in disability. Based on tools developed by Crombie (1996), the CRD developed forms to appraise studies that used single subject experimental designs, case studies and qualitative research. With further exploration, the CRD used appraisal forms with instructions developed by Law *et al.* (1998).

Between 2001 and 2003, each therapy discipline investigated the research evidence relating to one question of clinical relevance. All therapy staff were involved in the process of reviewing and critically appraising the literature, co-ordinated by research seniors and supported by the manager. SLTs examined the factors that affected the participation of children who use augmentative and alternative communication in school settings (Guidera *et al.*, 2002). Occupational therapists developed practice guidelines regarding facilitating play in children with physical disability following a critical appraisal of the literature by Murchland and colleagues (2003). Physiotherapists appraised the evidence for the use of Gross Motor Function Measure (GMFM-88) as a functional outcome measure for children with cerebral palsy and found that it was reliable and valid tool (Gibson and Physiotherapy Staff, 2001). Since the EBP tasks were undertaken as part of the clinicians' work, it took between 18 months and 3 years to gather and synthesize the evidence and to utilize it in clinical practice.

In the process of appraising the evidence for EBP, Novita staff were given the opportunity to provide feedback about perceived benefits and challenges. They identified that investigating the evidence gave them the opportunity to explore and discuss their understanding of key concepts in their disciplines and work practices through critical appraisal. This was seen to be extremely beneficial, and to help clinicians to update their knowledge and share this with families thus facilitating family-centred practice. Clinicians also identified a number of challenges, and recommendations for the future of the initiative, including:

- training was essential, and needed to start at a basic level of understanding, with small group sessions for following the various EBP steps
- appraisal of articles took time, and staff priorities for clinical service provision and organizational activities influenced the diligence of staff in reviewing research articles
- it was essential to have clear guidelines to support staff to approach the appraisal process, as confidence and competence of therapists in understanding the research impacted on the quality of appraisal

- compiling results of the appraisals was a challenge that would be helped by an efficient data management programme
- implementation of evidence / knowledge transfer to potentially alter practice takes time and requires a managed approach that includes ongoing education, support and follow-up.

Reflections on collaborative working

Novita is a unique organization that invests in research capacity by establishing its own CRD. Clients and families are aware that Novita is committed to ensuring that they have access to the current and best available interventions. Staff are encouraged and supported to develop and expand their research skills and to become critical reviewers. While the establishment of a CRD comes at a cost in terms of training, support and specialist staff, the outcomes continue to lead to a solid research foundation for clinical service provision.

Our success resulted in an increasing number of ideas being submitted by Novita staff and opportunities for collaboration with researchers from other agencies. Many of the research outcomes were incorporated or influenced the 2006–2010 Strategic Direction of the organization. For example, one project evaluating Novita's family-centred practice model (Raghavendra et al., 2007), highlighted the need for the organization to provide general information around disability issues to families.

One of the main benefits of the initiative has been the development of a research culture of critically questioning practices and asking about evidence. Further, research ideas have been developed that are clinically driven, facilitating investigation of the efficacy for interventions and understanding of issues around disability. In terms of challenges, we noted that a lack of adequate time and funding to conduct or complete research (including appropriate dissemination) was a problem. Clinicians had varying knowledge and skills in understanding research methodology and critical appraisal of research. It was also difficult to manage the increase in the number of research projects and thus the many requests of families and clients to participate in research. For example, we found that the ever growing number of projects has resulted in project outcomes not being developed for publication and outcomes not being translated into practice systematically. This is being addressed by establishing two strategic areas of research focus for the next three years, employing staff with research skills, implementing knowledge brokering and translation strategies such as developing easy to read summaries of projects, and continuing to involve clinicians in the research process.

The development of a successful CRD is dependent on many factors, and we feel that the following have made it possible to implement this model at Novita:

- Recognition of the importance of research, and support provided by the Novita Children's Services Board, the Chief Executive and senior management
- An organization-wide focus on high quality service delivery
- A research manager with formal qualifications in research, with clinical and research experience
- A high level of involvement and support provided by clinical managers of allied health disciplines

- The development of joint research/clinical senior therapist positions
- The involvement of families in research projects, and in the process of project selection (via involvement in the Clinical Research Subcommittee)
- Links with external agencies including university departments, hospital and the children's education sector to support and promote the generation of research ideas and the transfer of knowledge into practice.

With these factors in place, the CRD model has been sustained for nearly ten years, and the model has continued to develop and change over time. The benefits and challenges of the clinician–researcher model, and input from a range of external and internal stakeholders including families and clients of Novita are shaping the development of a new Division of Research and Innovation, and helping to identify research priorities. It is envisaged that Novita will continue to generate and translate knowledge to enhance the lives of children with disabilities and their families as well as provide opportunities and support for clinicians to develop their expertise in providing EBP.

Acknowledgements

The significant contributions made by Research Senior Therapists Sonya Murchland, Susan Gibson, Angela Guidera, Kylie Opperman and Violetta Hodges are acknowledged. Thanks to Clinical Managers of Allied Health, Catherine Olsson, Terry Lyons, Judy Sprod and Dr. Tim Connell for their leadership and enthusiasm for research and to Wendy Wake-Dyster, Director of Client Programs, for her ongoing support.

References

Baxter, P. (2008) Research priorities: Bless thee! Thou art translated. *Developmental Medicine & Child Neurology*, **50**, 323.

Blackstone, S. (2007) Knowledge translation. *Augmentative Communication News*, **19** (3), 2.

Crombie, I. (1996) *The Pocket Guide to Critical Appraisal: A Handbook for Health Care Professionals*. London: BMJ Publishing Group.

Gibson, S. and Physiotherapy Staff (2001) What is the evidence for the use of the gross motor function measure (GMFM-88) as a functional outcome measure for children with cerebral palsy? In *Novita Children's Services Research Report January 1999– June 2004* (p. 46). Adelaide, South Australia: Novita Children's Services.

Grace, E. (2004) School vocabulary in typically developing 6 year old Australian children. Honours thesis, Flinders University, South Australia.

Guidera, A., Raghavendra, P. and Olsson, C. (2002) Participation of users in school setting: research evidence. Paper presented at the Proceedings of the 10th Biennial Conference of the International Society for Augmentative and Alternative Communication, Odense, Denmark.

King, G., Currie, M., Smith, L., Servais, M. and McDougall, J. (2008) A framework of operating models for interdisciplinary research programs in clinical service organisations. *Evaluation and Program Planning*, **31**, 160–173.

Law, M., Stewart, D., Pollock, N., Letts, L., Bosch, J. and Westmorland, M. (1998) Occupational Therapy Evidence-based Practice Group. Retrieved July 9, 2008 from http://www.srs-mcmaster.ca/nbspnbspResearchResourcesnbspnbsp/ CentreforEvidenceBasedRehabilitation/EvidenceBasedPracticeResearchGroup/ tabid/630/Default.aspx

Manson, P., Guidera, A. and Raghavendra, P. (2000) Can preschool children learn the meaning of picture symbols without structured teaching? Paper presented at the Australian Cerebral Palsy Association Conference, 2000.

McGregor, S. (2007) Participation profiles of adolescents with and without complex communication needs: The relationship between social networks, communication and activity engagement. Honours thesis, Flinders University, South Australia.

Murchland, S. and Occupational Therapy Staff (2003) Evidence-based practice review of occupational therapy interventions to assist pre-school children with physical disabilities to become spontaneous and independent players and guidelines for clinical practice. In *Novita Children's Services Research Report January 1999–June 2004* (p. 16). Adelaide, South Australia: Novita Children's Services.

Olsson, C. (2003) The EBP experiences of an AAC service provider: diving in deep. *Perspectives on Augmentative and Alternative Communication [Newsletter of Division 12 Special Interest Group of the American Speech-Language-Hearing Association]*, 12, 15–19.

Raghavendra, P., Murchland, S., Bentley, M., Wake-Dyster, W. and Lyons, T. (2007) Parents' and service providers' perceptions of family-centred practice in a community based, paediatric disability service in Australia. *Child: Care, Health & Development*, 33 (5), 586–592.

12

Valuing evidence-based practice in the clinical setting – a showcase event

Siân E. Davies[1] and Tracey C. Dean[2]

[1]Principal Speech and Language Therapist, NHS East Lancashire, UK
[2]Manager of Speech and Language Therapy Services, NHS East Lancashire, UK

East Lancashire, in the north-west of England, covers five boroughs which include urban and rural economies, with areas of high levels of deprivation, and ethnic minority populations. The National Health Service (NHS) East Lancashire speech and language therapy service (and its predecessors) is part of the UK NHS and offers a comprehensive range of services to children and adults with a variety of clinical conditions, including learning difficulties. The service has an open referral system and is free at the point of care.

The authors are senior clinicians/managers within the service and have been in post for a significant period of time. Although evidence-based practice (EBP) is considered to be the responsibility of all clinicians, the lead is shared across the management team who regularly review how clinical practice is influenced by the evidence. From the 1990s onwards significant professional and political changes made it necessary to formalize the process in order to demonstrate the service's compliance.

In 1991 the Royal College of Speech and Language Therapists produced 'Communicating Quality' (RCSLT, 1991) a seminal text outlining standards for speech and language therapists (SLTs). This text marked a new era for the profession and led to recognition by SLTs of the need to develop the evidence base for interventions. The text was revised twice (in 1996 and 2006) to reflect changes in the evidence base, national strategic direction, legislative requirements and technologies but it still remains fundamental to the delivery of quality services to clients. The information in Communicating Quality (RCSLT, 2006) is supported by the 'Clinical Guidelines' (RCSLT, 2005) which collate for SLTs the current evidence base for interventions.

In 1997 a change in government in the UK resulted in a review of the NHS and significant changes to the way that it operated. The government laid out its vision in 'Clinical Governance: Quality in the new NHS' (Department of Health, 1999). It focused on the quality of the service and introduced the concept of clinical governance:

A framework through which NHS organisations are accountable for continuously improving the quality of their services and safeguarding high standards of care by creating an environment in which excellence in clinical care will flourish (p. 6).

Clinical governance placed the onus on services to:

- demonstrate that they were doing the most good and the least harm for the most number of people
- find out what works best and do it every time
- demonstrate that interventions have a sound evidence base.

The NHS East Lancashire SLT service embraced the concept of clinical governance and developed a strategy based on the premise that clinical governance is everyone's business. A key principle was that clinical governance should be integral to the way all staff think and act. However, the SLT service leaders recognized that in order to be able to provide evidence of governance activity, it would need to raise staff awareness of what they were already involved in that contributed to the clinical governance agenda as well as considering developments.

Strategies for creating an evidence-based culture in our service

Staff were familiar with some aspects of evaluating clinical practice. For example, they had experience in the use of audit to examine clinical and cost effectiveness. On the other hand, there were variable skill levels relating to utilizing evidence and to demonstrating the link between the evidence base and their own clinical practice. A challenge was therefore to develop a culture of embedding EBP within routine speech and language therapy practice, in a way that acknowledged and valued the experience and learning of staff who might feel threatened by the new culture. An additional key concern was to limit any additional work needed to meet the demands of clinical governance.

Rather than imposing the need for EBP, it was felt that a culture change would be achieved more effectively if the evidence base was made more accessible to staff so that it filtered into practice and staff were empowered to feel able to contribute to the evidence base for the profession. Developing the new culture of EBP should come from existing practice and continued professional development activities and these approaches should be fully integrated into everyday custom and practice. By taking small incremental steps and having some mandatory elements to get it started, it was hoped to give motivated staff something to build upon, while enabling others to take something on board which would act as a springboard for change.

In order to achieve this, a number of strategies were introduced.

- All staff received training on grades of evidence and critical appraisal skills. This training became a mandatory element of the induction programme for all new staff. The training was used as an opportunity to enable staff to identify learning objectives for their continued professional development activities to evaluate their learning in a more structured manner.

- Protected reading time was introduced as a means of encouraging staff to book time specifically to 'research' the evidence base in a particular area.
- All clinical staff were asked to produce an annual report which critically appraised a new piece of research in their clinical area.
- Discussions at team clinical meetings were more focused on EBP and critical appraisal.

In addition, a number of activities were developed to support integration of EBP into the service. These included developing evidence-based clinical pathways and caseload management documents and redefining the role of the service's lead clinicians to reinforce their responsibility for searching and evaluating emerging evidence. The establishment of a secondment post to The University of Manchester and the development of a specialist academic–clinical aphasia clinic further enhanced access to contemporary research and formed part of the strategy to support staff in undertaking research activity.

The Professional Development Forum

The initiatives and activities above led to significant cultural change. However, a need was identified for a means of acknowledging the value of what staff were doing, and of promoting role models which others could emulate. An 'event' to showcase EBP was developed in order to:

- develop staff confidence in their work in relation to EBP
- raise the profile of clinician-led research and act as a showcase for activities the service was engaged in
- enable staff to share information and learning with colleagues from very different areas of speech and language therapy.

The Professional Development Forum is a half day annual conference, which was established seven years ago as a showcase event for sharing and publicizing good practice within the SLT service. As the culture of both the profession and the service has changed, it has developed an increasing focus on EBP. It provides valuable time for reflection and sharing, on a personal, team and service-wide basis. All elements of the service are included which creates an important avenue for fostering cohesion across the teams.

Elements of the Professional Development Forum

Each Forum has a theme which is identified by the senior SLT team in advance and is influenced by current events and activities. Examples of themes have included:

- application of clinical guidelines and critical appraisal of literature to develop new ways of delivering services
- international influences, reflecting oversees visits, conferences, collaborations

---

> **Box 12.1   Example of presentations and posters showcased at the Professional Development Forum**
>
> Presentations:
>
> - A multi-centre randomized control trial evaluating effectiveness of speech and language therapy post acute stroke.
> - A combined therapy and drug treatment single case study.
> - Impact of a literature search in treatment, e.g. for a lady with learning difficulties and dysphagia.
> - Developing a fluency care pathway.
> - Use of an electronic whiteboard and software in running paediatric groups.
> - Changing roles – working within the classroom.
>
> Posters:
>
> - Accessible communication in schools.
> - School entry therapy.
> - Swallowing training packs for nursing homes.
> - Use of Jabadao (music-based intervention) with clients with learning difficulties.

- improved practice as reported against 'Standards for Better Health' (Department of Health, 2006)
- facilitating and collaborating in research.

The Forum has two components – presentations and poster displays. All staff, regardless of grade or levels of experience, are expected to contribute, either as individuals or as teams. Newly qualified practitioners display posters of their undergraduate project/dissertation.

For staff, the event provides an opportunity to develop presentation and display skills and to get peer feedback, whilst learning from colleagues and increasing their awareness of other initiatives in the service. The nature of the topics covered, together with minimizing the workload demands for the contributions, supports an ethos of EBP as part of 'routine' clinical activity.

Presentations are diverse, and range from formal clinical research projects, to the development of clinical pathways and the impact of evidence on therapy. Poster presentations are similarly diverse and support clinicians to understand the evidence about particular topics. See Box 12.1 for examples of presentations and posters.

The event is mandatory for all clinical staff (SLTs and assistants) and is always held in December as part of a celebration of the service's achievements during the year. It begins with a reflection by the service manager on the key activities of the year, including achievement of targets against the service's performance framework. It is timed such that it ends with the annual Christmas meal. This combination of a formal showcasing of activity together with a social event at a natural juncture in the year seems to be a significant factor in establishing a successful mindset for the event. Senior managers from the organization are invited to the event as a way of promoting good practice at a wider level.

The impact of the Forum

Key themes emerge when staff are asked to reflect on the impact of the Forum. These key themes are:

- team building
- motivation and inspiration
- skill development.

Team building

Staff consistently identify that the Forum provides an opportunity for team building. They are able to network with other SLTs – especially across teams who rarely meet except at busy staff meetings. The Forum provides an opportunity for a less pressured and hurried approach, with plenty of time for chat and discussion. The preparation for the Forum creates positive rapport within teams as they meet to work together on presentations. Importantly, it provides a time of solidarity and celebration across the department.

The Forum supports an awareness of the work of other colleagues, seeing how their work is developing and changing. Staff are also made aware of the trends influencing developments and how the different parts of the service fit together, looking for areas of overlap and application to reduce duplication of workload and to extend practice.

Motivation and inspiration

Having the opportunity to present, and to hear about the work of others, is reported to be motivating and inspirational to staff. The Forum is 'positive time' – away from the nitty-gritty and business matters of other types of staff meetings and training events. It is a chance to focus on promoting the positive aspects of the service, rather than the challenges and difficulties. It is a time to feel proud about the high level of work going on in the service as a whole. A key element of the Forum is that it demonstrates that EBP is achievable through showing concrete examples; this makes it less of an abstract concept. Staff also report that it is valuable to have a summary of the year as evidence of how the service is growing and developing.

Skill development

The Forum presents an opportunity for staff to practise presentation skills in front of a supportive and sympathetic audience and generate materials that can be re-used at other training and promotional events. Staff can see the impact of different presentation and display styles, for example, videos, case studies, lighter topics and more theoretical discussions, in an informal and relaxed atmosphere. By listening and learning about others' EBP activities, the event is a Continuing Professional Development (CPD) opportunity and contributes to the number of CPD hours required by the Royal College of Speech and Language Therapists and the Health Professions Council.

We find that these three themes are consistent, regardless of whether the staff commenting are newly qualified, new to the service, or staff who have been employed by the service since before the initiative developed. This suggests that it meets both individual and collective needs and that these are needs of staff throughout their careers.

Although the event is one that has been positively received in the main, there were a number of barriers to be overcome in its development. Staff initially viewed the Forum as 'something extra you have to do' but this has diminished over time as the need for a clinical evidence base is a more common expectation. Some staff saw their activity around EBP as routine and therefore were reluctant to share it with others, especially if the practice was not 'gold standard'. With encouragement and familiarity this has improved but it still remains a difficulty for some staff. Practical barriers included the need for information technology skills and resources for the presentations but over time these have been overcome. A more recent issue has been how to deal with the competition and rivalry that has now started to develop between and within teams. This is being managed by ensuring the pro-gramme offers equal opportunities to different clinical areas and by managing carefully the expectations of the presenters.

Key to the ongoing success of the Forum is ensuring the appropriate amount of time and support is made available for the presentation/display preparation. Importantly, the initiative is supported by senior management which is essential in a large and growing organization, especially when there is tension between the need to develop EBP and celebrate achievement, as well as to address waiting times and meet targets. This support needs to be evident at the managerial level to both facilitate and affirm the activity. A key finding of Pennington *et al.* (2005) was that management commitment and support was associated with increased adherence to clinical guidelines, and that the department where the SLT worked influenced their use of research. Where services are divided into teams (in our case four clinical teams), the complexity and diversity of services can lead to working in silos, without appreciating or benefiting from the experience of others. Cross-team discussions providing different perspectives lead us to function much more as one profession and promotes the importance of sharing work that others can benefit from; for example, symbol communication systems used in schools influencing aphasia rehabilitation; acute dysphagia screening in hospital influencing a residential unit. The commitment has to be ongoing as staff con-stantly change so what has become a routine activity for some is a new initiative for others.

Reflections on the Professional Development Forum into the future

Review and change are a key part of an initiative such as this and some areas currently under consideration include the following.

- Building in more time for viewing posters. One suggestion is to replace them with an e-document to look at after the event.
- Rethinking presentation times, as there is currently a perception that there are too many presentations with not enough time per presentation.
- Supporting less experienced staff in their presentation skills.

- Supporting staff to make real changes on the basis of what they learn in the Forum. It's easy to attend and enjoy but not really change one's own practice.

As this showcase event is now well established, there is a need to extend its aims as clinical governance and EBP have become more firmly embedded in the NHS and the service and the expectations of new graduates are that this is routine activity. As it has evolved, the emerging themes have become more focused and more closely tied to the service work plan to enable it to more formally be part of the cycle of review and planning. With improvements in information technology, the material from the event is electronically stored on shared access facilities and this serves as a permanent archive. It is also hoped that there will be some publications. However, whilst these innovations are exciting and forward thinking, it is important that the routine, everyday, sound grassroots practice is not marginalized – this is at the core of SLT services and needs to be equally valued.

A significant challenge ahead is how to share the evidence base being developed with a wider audience. Changes in commissioning of NHS services mean that the evidence base is being requested both for development bids and to demonstrate the effectiveness of funding. The increased involvement of clients in developing services will enable them to contribute to determining the direction of evidence-based activity and our vision would be to include them in the showcasing and celebration of the service's achievements in the future.

Acknowledgements

The authors would like to acknowledge the ongoing commitment and enthusiasm of the speech and language therapy staff of NHS East Lancashire for evidence-based practice.

References

Department of Health (1999) *Clinical Governance: Quality in the New NHS (HSC 1999/065)*. London: DH.

Department of Health (2006) *Standards for Better Health*. London: DH.

Pennington, L., Roddam, H., Burton, C., Russell, I., Godfrey, C. and Russell, D. (2005) Promoting research use in speech and language therapy: a cluster randomized controlled trial to compare the clinical effectiveness and costs of two training strategies. *Clinical Rehabilitation*, **19**, 387–397.

Royal College of Speech and Language Therapists (1991) *Communicating Quality* (1st edn). London: RCSLT.

Royal College of Speech and Language Therapists (1996) *Communicating Quality* (2nd edn). London: RCSLT.

Royal College of Speech and Language Therapists (2005) *Clinical Guidelines*. Oxon: Speechmark.

Royal College of Speech and Language Therapists (2006) *Communicating Quality* (3rd edn). London: RCSLT.

13

Launching and sustaining an evidence-based highly specialist service

Sheena Round and Sarah Beazley

Consultant Speech and Language Therapists, Cheshire and Merseyside Network for Permanent Hearing Impairment, Liverpool Primary Care Trust, UK

In this chapter, we would like to share with you how our specialist clinical network came to the position it is in today, and how having this specialist service provides a context that promotes and supports evidence-based practice (EBP). We will consider some of the matters that we are wrestling with in the current political, financial, economic and social climate. We hope that you will be able to see some similarities to your own area of expertise that will either make you feel better about your own situation or inspire you to set something similar in motion.

Networks are growing in number in the National Health Service (NHS) in the UK and at the time of writing, the NHS web site (www.networks.nhs.uk) lists over 500 networks 'which may be formal, informal, clinical, professional, leadership, geographical, theme or specialty based'. It is intended that these networks achieve some form of 'collective efficiency' (Bessant and Tsekouras, 2001).

The highly specialist clinical network described in this chapter was designed to cover the UK region of Cheshire and Merseyside, which has a mixed rural and urban population of 2.4 million. The network exists to ensure that every person who is deaf has access to a highly specialist speech and language therapist (SLT) and to provide specialist support for the users of the service, including both individuals and their families/carers.

Why and how did the network start?

Prior to the implementation of the network, access to specialist SLT support for deaf people was something of a 'postcode lottery' in Cheshire and Merseyside. Many deaf children and adults received no SLT service at all whilst others saw a local SLT who may or may not have had additional training in working with deaf people and who could not cross Primary Care Trust (PCT) boundaries. Where money was made available for a highly specialist service for deaf people, recruitment was difficult; if appointed the SLT could feel isolated professionally, retention was often problematic and finance for the post was then sometimes reallocated. This reflected the national picture reported by Evans and Robinshaw in 1999. They found that 46% of SLT managers had no structured preschool service for hearing impaired children in contrast to the education sector, where services existed in all cases.

Obviously, this situation did not meet the needs of service users, nor did it enable evidence-based care. In our region, parents, professionals and a local Member of Parliament began campaigning for a service that:

- gave equal access to a highly specialist SLT for all deaf people across the region
- used a care pathway that functioned in the context of the other services provided for deaf people and their families.

The outcome was a commissioned two-year project to identify the SLT input that would be needed and to develop a possible care pathway, with contributions from other professionals and parents.

Setting up the network: reviewing the evidence

We needed to consider how best to provide an equitable, responsive SLT service across the region. In this context, a research project was undertaken (Round, 2005) to understand the experiences of users of the service, specifically those with a cochlear implant (an inner ear electronic hearing device). As part of the project, an evaluation of the literature about the delivery of regional specialist services was conducted. This revealed the following themes:

- The service should be centred on the service users, not the professionals (White and Featherstone, 2005)
- Families wanted a co-ordinated service that shared information between professionals (Abbot et al., 2005).

The cochlear implant service users participating in the project expressed the desire to:

- access resources locally (adults and children)
- be in contact with child-friendly staff
- be seen in a child-friendly environment.

A further source of evidence was from local experts representing health, education and social services. Through formal and informal discussions, these professionals indicated the need for flexibility across PCT boundaries; close multiagency working; and cover for absences.

We recognized that the number of therapists needed for the population in question would be driven partly by 'numbers' and also by our initial network focus on developing a service for children. The published epidemiological evidence (Fortnum and Davis, 1997; Fortnum et al., 2001) indicated that the incidence of permanent childhood hearing impairment for hearing losses over 40 dB is fairly static at 1.1 per 1000 live births rising by 50–90% by the age of nine. A stable incidence meant that we could use prevalence data provided by audiology departments across the region. This gave an indication of the number of bilaterally severely-profoundly deaf children and adolescents in the area to be covered by the network both at the time (a total of 395 children and adolescents) and in the future.

Enderby and Davies (1989) discussed the need to consider both demand and also treatment evaluation when thinking about caseload numbers. We had to consider how many days of an SLT's time would be needed for the 'existing' caseload from the prevalence figures for each PCT (the demand). We also took into account professional consensus, and consideration of the potential care pathway (treatment evaluation). Caseloads were set at 50 for the full-time highly specialist SLTs across the region.

From evidence to practice

Network approaches are well established in the NHS but none existed for this specialty. We still had a series of questions about the potential service to consider.

- How was this service to be delivered in a responsive way over such a wide geographical area? Flexible job descriptions would be needed, in order to allow SLTs to cross PCT boundaries.
- Recruitment of specialists would be difficult. We knew that this would mean training SLTs as it was unlikely that we could recruit the skilled staff needed. In the field of working with deaf people, there are established post-qualification courses, mostly requiring travel to London. As access to these courses might be impractical for individual therapists from our region, we needed a different approach to training to meet our geographical constraints and also to provide more work-based learning.
- What could a care pathway look like? We knew that it would need to follow the service users' journey from referral to discharge, acknowledging the input of the other professionals already assisting deaf people and their families. This would have many advantages including setting the SLT provision in the context of other services and creating a framework to collect regional audit data.

In order to begin developing the network, meetings were set up with heads of the various professional groups, families and voluntary groups to discuss a virtual care pathway for a team that didn't yet exist. These meetings were approached positively by health service managers but often treated guardedly by heads of other services. It soon became clear that one of the main reasons for this was that the project was instigated by health rather than jointly commissioned across sectors.

There is much evidence in the literature about the barriers to integrated working such as competing priorities and unpooled resources (Hannigan, 1997). Cohesiveness amongst different professionals depends on the agreed parameters for co-operation (Easen *et al.*, 2000) and in the developmental phase of the network, such aspects were not particularly well established.

In line with current thinking (Department for Children, Schools and Families, 2008), we continued to explore more fruitful ways to ensure collaborative working. One example of this is joint professional training, and therapy groups. Joint training has been identified as one way to facilitate inter-professional practice (O'Toole and Kirkpatrick, 2007). We have developed multiagency training days and both family and professional feedback has been positive. We have also run social communication groups jointly with assistance from other professionals, learning support assistant training packages and also early communication groups for parents. The critical mass of highly specialist SLTs has meant that we can devise and host such courses more easily.

Inevitably, there have been other adjustments in the network in response to changing social, economic and political parameters as well as to our own increasing confidence as a team. Five years later, we remain a strong but flexible group led by the two of us, with 11 highly specialist and one principal therapist.

How the network supports EBP

We have found that the network provides a service delivery model that supports EBP in a range of different ways. We will focus here on how it does this in relation to training, to family focused service delivery and to the balance between direct and indirect therapy.

The network supports evidence-based training

We use an evidence-based approach centred on the Knowledge and Skills Framework (Department of Health, 2004) in order to take an SLT three to four years post-qualification to starting to function at highly specialist level. This approach focuses on providing evidence that learning has been implemented in the workplace. This occurs via documentation and through recorded discussions of research projects and clinical cases during supervision sessions provided by the network consultants.

The network supports therapists to be more family focused

The importance of placing families (Carter *et al.*, 2007) and children (Watson *et al.*, 2007) centrally to any planning about their lives is a significant theme in the NHS and as a network we support therapists in being flexible in their approach to working with families. For example, we designed network services around home visits for pre-schoolers in response to the suggestion for child-friendly environments (Round, 2005) but we are finding that some families prefer to be seen elsewhere such as in a children's centre. Part of our ongoing commitment to becoming family-led is the development of more frequent and comprehensive opportunities for service users to make decisions around service delivery. We are developing a range of ways that children can comment and for example have found that the use of 'video diaries' at the summer schools have been a popular and effective way to enable reflection on the service.

The network supports the evidence base around the role of SLTs

Although SLTs still carry out direct therapy, many are moving towards an increasingly consultative role (Law *et al.*, 2002). As a network, we need to ensure that consultative working is an additional part of the highly specialist SLT's skill set. The evidence base for this approach may initiate a different way of working but its effectiveness for this client group still needs to be monitored via outcomes in terms of skill acquisition and feedback questionnaires for users and their families.

The network supports evidence-based reflection

We collected some evidence from the therapists about their experience of working in the network, using questionnaires. All therapists thought that the network had a positive influence on their relationship with families and with staff in other agencies. One hundred per cent also thought that working in the network had increased the effectiveness of their practice, and that the network had enabled them to access appropriate training. In addition, the therapists indicated where the network needed more direction and clarity suggesting, for example, that we need to formalize a process for identifying which therapists have done which assessments with clients, to avoid reduplication. Such data enables the network to respond to those who work within it and improve the work environment of the staff.

Developing the evidence base further

We recognize that there is an obligation as the network becomes more established, to add to the specialist evidence base in a range of different ways. There is an expectation of all our SLTs to be research active in some way as specified in the NHS descriptors of the advanced therapist job profile (National Health Service, 2008).

Provan and Brinton Milward (2001) discuss the complexity of evaluating the effectiveness of networks and we are aware that gathering evidence will be a multifaceted and ongoing process. Working with a university-based researcher, we are looking at ways to carry out ongoing full service evaluation. This aims to include feedback from service users and other professionals across the agencies locally including Children's Hearing Services Working Groups. The service evaluation will also involve voluntary agencies, commissioners and cochlear implant teams. We will continue to monitor responses from the network therapists and also other SLTs from neighbouring PCTs who have been able to use the network resource to develop individual highly specialist training packages.

Within this plan, we also aim to cultivate an evidence-led culture including supporting individual highly specialist SLTs in carrying out research, widening our use of expert consensus to back up our work as well as the use of systematic reviews and experimental studies. We propose to use the network framework to enable us to carry out multiple baseline case studies exploring particular patterns and approaches to add to the specialist knowledge base.

Reflections on the specialist network

As a model, the network has proved to be successful in terms of core outcomes; every person who is deaf in the region has access to a highly specialist SLT who is well trained and supported, recruitment and retention of staff is no longer an issue and staff can move flexibly across PCT boundaries.

If the network stayed the same it would stagnate, not necessarily being fit for purpose for the next and following decades as technology advances and the shape of services change. This is where research, commissioning and clinical practice as an interactive and continuous process must be the template for an effective, high quality network.

The evidence base helped to form the network originally and now, in turn, the network is contributing to that knowledge base in order to inform and facilitate future service development. It has evolved to a model of care where commissioners and clinicians continue to share expertise and knowledge including current research evidence in order to develop services for deaf people on an ongoing basis.

References

Abbot, D., Watson, D. and Townsley, R. (2005) The proof of the pudding: what difference does multi-agency working make to families with disabled children with complex health care needs? *Child and Family Social Work*, **10** (3), 229–238.

Bessant, J. and Tsekouras, G. (2001) Developing learning networks. *AI and Society*, **15** (1–2), 82–98.

Carter, B., Cummings, J. and Cooper, L. (2007) An exploration of best practice in multi-agency working and the experiences of families of children with complex health needs. What works well and what needs to be done to improve practice for the future? *Journal of Clinical Nursing*, **16** (3), 527–539.

Department for Children, Schools and Families (2008) *Children's Trusts: statutory guidance on inter-agency cooperation to improve the wellbeing of children, young people and their families*. London: DCSF.

Department of Health (2004) *The NHS Knowledge and Skills Framework (NHS KSF) and the development review process* [Publication No. DH_4009176]. London: DH.

Easen, P., Atkins, M. and Dyson, A. (2000) Inter-professional collaboration and conceptualisations of practice. *Children and Society*, **14**, 335–367.

Enderby, P. and Davies, P. (1989) Communication disorders: Planning a service to meet the needs. *International Journal of Language and Communication Disorders*, **24** (3), 301–331.

Evans, R. and Robinshaw, H. (1999) *Service provision for preschool deaf children: Report to The Nuffield Foundation June 1999*. Uxbridge, UK: Brunel University College.

Fortnum, H. and Davis, A. (1997) Epidemiology of permanent childhood hearing impairment in Trent region 1985–1993. *British Journal of Audiology*, **31** (6), 409–446.

Fortnum, H.M., Summerfield, A.Q., Marshall, D.H., Davis, A.C. and Bamford, J.M. (2001) Prevalence of permanent childhood hearing impairment in the United Kingdom and implications for universal neonatal hearing screening questionnaire based ascertainment study. *British Medical Journal*, **323**, 1–6.

Hannigan, B. (1997) Joint working in community mental health: prospects and challenges. *Health and Social Care in the Community*, **7** (1), 25–31.

Law, J., Lindsay, G., Peacey, N., *et al.* (2002) Consultation as a model for providing speech and language therapy in schools: a panacea or one step too far? *Child Language Teaching and Therapy*, **18** (2), 145–163.

National Health Service (2008) National profiles for speech and language therapists. Retrieved 7 October 2009, from http://www.nhsemployers.org/pay-conditions/pay-conditions-1988.cfm

O'Toole, C. and Kirkpatrick, V. (2007) Building collaboration between professionals in health and education through interdisciplinary training. *Child Language Teaching and Therapy*, **23** (3), 325–352.

Provan, K. and Brinton Milward, H. (2001) Do networks really work? A framework for evaluating public-sector organizational networks. *Public Administration Review*, **61** (4), 414–423.

Round, S. (2005) What are the views of cochlear implant users and their carers concerning the services provided. Unpublished Masters thesis, Department of Healthcare Studies, Manchester Metropolitan University, Manchester.

Watson, D., Abbott, D. and Townsley, R. (2007) Listen to me, too! Lessons from involving children with complex healthcare needs in research about multi-agency services. *Child: Care, Health and Development*, **33** (1), 90–95.

White, S. and Featherstone, B. (2005) Communicating misunderstandings: multi-agency work as social practice. *Child and Family Social Work*, **10** (3), 207–216.

14

Strategic approaches to promoting the value of EBP (commentary on Section Three)

Hazel Roddam and Jemma Skeat

The chapters in this section have delivered insights into a wide range of strategic approaches that have helped to support speech and language therapists (SLTs) to embed a more evidence-based approach across all aspects of their service delivery. In particular they have highlighted ways in which the value of evidence-based practice (EBP) can be communicated to staff within an SLT team, as well as across a wider organization, plus externally to other stakeholders and our service users. These contributors have shared their own experiences of leadership, through which they have sought to influence others with their vision and values, to promote EBP and to support staff to work in new ways. The ways in which these individuals have motivated and inspired their staff and colleagues has echoed through each chapter.

Through reflecting on the initiatives described in these chapters, a number of common strands have emerged including: promoting a questioning and learning approach; promoting the value of EBP; creating ownership by active engagement of all staff in service planning; and bridging the research–practice gap by increasing clinicians' confidence that it is possible for them to embed research into their practice. These contributions have shown how simple initiatives have the potential to motivate and inspire staff, for example the annual event described by Siân and Tracey as a 'springboard for change' (p. 88).

Another clear theme is that this is necessarily an iterative, ongoing process: we cannot be complacent as we will need to constantly assure ourselves as well as our stakeholders that our SLT services remain fit for purpose, in line with the most current evidence for services that are both clinically effective as well as cost effective. This is clearly articulated by Sheena and Sarah in relation to their highly specialized service. It is essential that all staff perceive this iterative aspect of EBP to be a fundamental element of their professional identity, for the benefit of all their current and prospective service users; and that it is not perceived to be an externally-imposed, and therefore less meaningful, requirement.

We would like, in this short commentary, to consider two aspects of embedding EBP into the 'culture' of SLT departments and/or organizations. One is the use of 'champions' and other agents for change. The other is measuring culture – how will we know when we are 'EBP ready'?

Identifying and supporting agents for change

A number of our contributed chapters throughout the book have illustrated that it is not only service managers who have the potential to positively influence colleagues in relation to EBP. The idea of using 'champions' for EBP (in order to promote the dissemination of research findings, and to support training in EBP skills) has been suggested as one way of providing EBP leadership in clinical practice. Some have suggested that these could be in the form of experienced outreach workers or facilitators who would visit departments to work alongside staff (Tse *et al.*, 2004; Pennington *et al.*, 2005). However, this requires access to allied health professional (AHP) staff who are themselves appropriately experienced in implementing research findings in their own clinical practice, and this may prove to be difficult. Individuals who additionally possess other qualities and traits as effective opinion leaders could prove to be exceptionally rare (Thompson *et al.*, 2001). We would like to highlight that students and recently qualified clinicians often have considerable energy and enthusiasm as well as valuable skills to share with colleagues, and can be effective 'champions' in their own way. The chapters in Section Two have illustrated that the new generation of SLTs may have a firmer foundation for EBP than those who have been practicing for many years, and it is important that this is not only nurtured but is allowed to inspire and encourage others. Parimala's chapter in this section also showcases champions for EBP in the form of dual clinical–research roles that are embedded in allied health departments. These types of roles may provide local access to EBP skills and knowledge, and this is one approach that may support evidence-based decision-making at the point of clinical care, as well as facilitating clinical research. There are some specific recommendations around change agents which we would like to briefly highlight. Harvey *et al.* (2002) and Stetler (2003) both argued that dedicated roles are needed – that is, people should have the nominated task of facilitating or supporting EBP, and this should not be a 'casual' thing that an interested person takes on in addition to all of their other duties. There is also a strong argument that the success of such roles is highly dependent on the active support of senior management within their organizations (Greenhalgh *et al.*, 2004).

The challenges of measuring a culture that supports EBP

In Chapter 3, we discussed the importance of individuals' attitudes towards EBP, and the influence of the workplace context was also highlighted in that section. It is an ongoing challenge to construct valid measures of the culture of teams and organizations (Baker, 1998). Siân and Tracey's chapter highlights the need for a meaningful indicator of the local 'ethos', which would support managers to identify strategic approaches (for example, in terms of their leadership style) and help to promote progress in embedding EBP across their local context.

One recent project has aimed to identify good practice in establishing an EBP approach in the UK specifically for AHP services, through benchmarking the relevant aspects of organizational context (Roddam *et al.*, 2007). An integrative review of key bodies of literature across healthcare services was conducted (French *et al.*, 2009) to identify key factors about the organization that would indicate its strategic capacity for promoting and supporting EBP. These factors comprise systems for the acquisition of new knowledge (absorptive capacity), as well as systems for knowledge sharing and knowledge use (receptive capacity). A self-evaluation questionnaire tool was subsequently constructed to allow teams (e.g. uniprofessional departments or multidisciplinary AHP services) to rate their EBP 'readiness'. The tool uses key statements against which each team rates their performance, supporting this with explicit justifications detailing recent local initiatives, systems or processes. The project outcomes (Roddam *et al.*, 2007) comprised comparative benchmark rankings, as well as extensive repositories of good practice exemplars, which were disseminated across the wider organization. Since this project, the prototype paper-based survey has been updated to an on-line version and has demonstrated excellent internal reliability. This tool is currently undergoing external validation, following which the authors hope that it can be made available to be used by SLTs and other AHPs in the future, in order to support embedding EBP. This project has additionally offered training and support to nominated Facilitators from each participating service, so that these individuals can undertake the role of EBP champion in their own workplace, based on the recommendations for dedicated roles (Harvey *et al.*, 2002; Stetler, 2003). The Facilitators have an additional responsibility to ensure that the feedback reports are translated into specified action plans. The project has generated significant insights into knowledge transfer processes in healthcare services and the team hopes to share these through future publications which are currently in preparation.

Summary

The importance of a supportive context for EBP cannot be over-emphasized. Even with the most skilled and enthusiastic SLTs possible, there are specific barriers that exist in our organizations and teams which can impede our ability to truly embed EBP. We hope that the diverse examples provided in this section will give you some ideas about ways that your team can support a positive EBP culture, whether this be through celebrating achievements, creating expectations through leadership, embedding positions or roles that provide practical support for EBP, or in other ways.

References

Baker, M. (1998) Taking the strategy forward. In M. Baker and S. Kirk (eds), *Research and Development for the NHS: Evidence, Evaluation and Effectiveness* (2nd edn). Oxford: Radcliffe Medical Press.

French, B., Thomas, L.H., Baker, P., Burton, C.R., Pennington, L. and Roddam, H. (2009) What can management theories offer evidence-based practice? A comparative analysis of measurement tools for organisational context. *Implementation Science*, **4**: 28. Retrieved 7 October from http://www.implementationscience.com/content/4/1/28

Greenhalgh, T., Robert, G., MacFarlane, F., Bate, P. and Kytiakidou, O. (2004) Diffusion of innovations in service organisations: systematic review and recommendations. *Millbank Quarterly*, **82** (4).

Harvey, G., Loftus-Hills, A., Rycroft-Malone, J., *et al*. (2002). Getting evidence into practice: the role and function of facilitation. *Journal of Advanced Nursing*, **37** (6), 577–588.

Pennington, L., Roddam, H., Burton, C., Russell, I., Russell, D. and Godfrey, C. (2005) Promoting research use in speech and language therapy: a cluster randomised controlled trial to compare the clinical effectiveness and costs of two training strategies. *Clinical Rehabilitation*, **19** (4), 387–397.

Roddam, H., Baker, P., Burton, C., Thomas, L.H., French, B. and Pennington, L. (2007) *Benchmarking for factors that promote evidence-based practice*. 27th World Congress of the Association of Logopedics and Phoniatrics, Copenhagen.

Stetler, C.B. (2003) The role of the organisation in translating research into evidence-based practice. *Outcomes Management*, **7** (3), 97–103.

Thompson, C., McCaughan, D., Cullum, N., Sheldon T., Mulhall, A. and Thompson, D.R. (2001) Research information in nurses' clinical decision-making: what is useful? *Journal of Advanced Nursing*, **36** (3), 376–388.

Tse, S., Lloyd, C., Penman, M., King, R. and Bassett, H. (2004) Evidence-based practice and rehabilitation: occupational therapy in Australia and New Zealand experiences. *International Journal of Rehabilitation Research*, **27** (4), 269–274.

Section Four

Making the evidence work for us

15

The importance of listening to the views of clients

Pirkko Rautakoski

Speech and Language Therapist, Senior Lecturer,
Åbo Akademi University, Turku, Finland

In this chapter I will explore how working in an evidence-based approach needs to take account clients own perceptions and preferences. I will start by describing why the views of clients are important, and will then explore how clients can be involved in setting goals, choosing interventions, and evaluating the effectiveness of interventions. Some specific examples, applying these ideas to areas of speech and language therapy practice, are included. My background of over 20 years of clinical work as a speech and language therapist (SLT) with adults with different communication disorders, and my research work in aphasia intervention, has guided my interest in the effectiveness of the interventions, and the need to include the views of clients.

Why involve clients?

The values and expectations of the clients are one of the three core strands of evidence-based practice. Therefore, person-centredness is a key part of being an evidence-based clinician. A person-centred approach, including listening carefully to client needs, is also a foundation principle of professionalism (Worrall, 2006). A framework for considering client perspectives is provided by International Classification of Functioning, Disability and Health (ICF) of the World Health Organization (2001). With the framework of ICF, the experiences of individuals with a variety of health concerns can better be described. The framework allows us not only to describe the limitations of persons with health concerns but also positive things, what activities they can do, how they can participate in their lives, and personal factors such as coping skills and attitudes. The ICF has widened perspectives within the field of disability and rehabilitation, and has contributed greatly to the shift from the traditional 'medical model' towards a social model, where client views are valued (Byng and Duchan, 2005).

In addition to these professional concerns, listening to clients may also impact on the effectiveness of therapy. There is a risk of poor outcomes for intervention if the goals of the clients and the speech and language therapists are in dissonance (Worrall, 2006). Clients who feel that they are heard may also perceive that their treatment is more effective, and achieve greater recovery (Byng *et al.*, 2002).

Involving clients in speech and language therapy

Person-centred goal-setting is one approach for attaining meaningful outcomes for people with communication disorders and their families (Worrall, 2006). SLTs long ago noticed that the medical model and impairment-level goals are too narrow. The aim of speech and language therapy intervention is not always to 'cure', but rather to improve function, reduce or limit disability, and improve wellbeing. To be effective, goal setting needs to be considered in wider, real-world context including more social issues (Byng *et al.*, 2002). Accordingly the clients' conceptions of their communication, therapy goals and the effects of the intervention should be taken into account (Parr and Byng, 2000; Worrall, 2006).

It has been shown that clients and SLTs value different things as a success in therapy (Morris *et al.*, 2004). Measuring changes in the symptoms and severity of the language disorder has very much been the way to measure the outcomes of speech and language therapy interventions. However, the ICF model also encourages a person-centred approach to the evaluation of services, including the perspective of the clients receiving the services (Kagan and Duchan, 2004). The framework emphasizes the evaluation of participation as well as body functions and activities. The insider perspective on one's own communication is essential because no other approach can provide this personal information (Eadie *et al.*, 2006).

Specific methods and measures that include client views

There are a number of tools and techniques that exist to evaluate user perspectives. The following sections are not intended to be an exhaustive list of existing work, but are some examples that may be feasible for use in clinical practice.

Overall Assessment of the Speaker's Experience of Stuttering (OASES)

The efficacy of stuttering treatment has usually been assessed with objective measures such as percentage of syllables stuttered. However, stuttering should be looked from a wider perspective and also take into account the disability and the handicap it causes (Yaruss, 1998). Adapting the new framework of ICF, Yaruss and Quesal (2006) have developed a measurement instrument for documenting stuttering treatment outcomes from a broader, person-centred perspective. This self-assessment method named Overall Assessment of the Speakers's Experience of Stuttering (OASES) includes components for evaluating the speaker's affective, behavioural, and cognitive reactions to stuttering in addition to assessing the consequences of stuttering in terms of observable behaviours, functional communication, and quality of life. Information about these real world consequences of stuttering helps clinicians to understand the broad nature of stuttering as a disorder but also to evaluate the outcomes of stuttering interventions.

Swallowing Quality of Life (SWAL-QOL)

Instrumental methods to examine clinical features of dysphagia have developed a great deal and they are an important part of diagnosis. However, also with this group the client's perspective, his/her quality of life and client satisfaction should be evaluated. McHorney *et al.* (2002) used clients' subjective and objective concerns about swallowing to develop a client-based, dysphagia-specific outcomes tool, the Swallowing Quality of Life (SWAL-QOL) and Swallowing Quality of Care (SWAL-CARE) to enhance information on treatment variations and treatment effectiveness.

Quality of life measures in voice therapy

When assessing the voice, objective and instrumental measures are often used. Additionally, many therapists use a multidimensional voice analysis protocol for monitoring voice intervention, including a structured questionnaire on voice problems in daily life (Behrmann, 2005). Voice disorders can have an impact on physical, mental, social, emotional, and communicative functions (Franic *et al.*, 2005). The result of Krischke *et al.*'s (2005) work supports the observation that voice disorders significantly influence clients' health-related quality of life (HRQL). A number of voice-disorder specific instruments have been developed to allow patients to evaluate their quality of life. Some examples are the Voice-Related Quality of Life (V-RQOL) (Hogikyan and Sethuraman, 1999) and the Voice Handicap Index (VHI) (Jacobson *et al.*, 1997). The VHI is a questionnaire measuring the impact of voice problems in daily life. It has been translated and validated in several languages and it is currently the most widely used quality of life instrument in the area.

Person-centred approaches for people with aphasia

It is in the field of aphasia that clinical SLTs and researchers have most strongly advocated the need to listen to the client and their carers. Maybe this is because aphasia is often a chronic difficulty; people with aphasia have to live with their aphasia. The aim of services should be to ensure the clients and their significant others are able to live healthily with communication disability (Byng *et al.*, 2002). However, this principle can be applied also with clients with other kinds of communication disorders and their significant others.

Up until the 1980s, the rehabilitation of people with aphasia was influenced by the traditional medical model. In the 1990s, the consequences the aphasia had on the person's life and psychosocial well-being was gradually considered (Kagan and Gailey, 1993; LeDorze and Brassard, 1995; Lyon *et al.*, 1997). The aim of rehabilitation became to reduce the disability and the barriers that the aphasia caused, and to improve the quality of life (Ramsberger, 1994). It was acknowledged that people with aphasia need, in addition to the linguistic interventions, rehabilitation that supports their ability to maintain social contacts and to rebuild their lives.

Alongside this there was growing interest in 'functional communication' – getting the message through by any communication means – and in the importance of the support of the communication partner (Holland, 1991; Kagan *et al.*, 2001; Kagan and Gailey, 1993; Lyon *et al.*, 1997). Therefore, the barriers that restricted the activity and the participation were no longer considered to arise only from the individual but also potentially from the environment – for example, inexperienced communication partners (Kagan, 1998; LeDorze and Brassard, 1995; Pound *et al.*, 2002).

Although the medical model and the impairment level goals still influence the work of SLTs to a great extent, in aphasiology there are many researchers and clinical SLTs who have as a leading philosophy in their work to involve the clients in setting the goals and evaluating the outcomes of the interventions (Chapey *et al.*, 2000; Worrall, 2000; Pound *et al.*, 2001). The social model of disability has led to more client-led approaches instead of objective and clinician-controlled approaches in evaluation of the benefits of therapy (Kagan and Duchan, 2004). The Life Participation Approach to Aphasia (LPAA) is a framework where client involvement is central because life participation is the explicit goal of treatment and the key area to be evaluated (Chapey *et al.*, 2000). Judgements about the success of the therapy are based on whether clients perceive positive changes in 'living with aphasia'. ICF and LPAA take into account the importance of treatment and evaluation related to coping with a disability rather than solely on curing it.

Obtaining the views of clients with communication disorders

To enable people with communication disorders to be able to actively participate in goal setting, choosing interventions and evaluating the outcomes of therapy require some special arrangements. Their perspectives may be hard to capture because of the linguistic problems. Most commonly used client-report methods are based on spoken or written language, and thus they are not accessible to people with severe communication problems (Sarno, 1997; Hilari and Byng, 2003). However, a variety of methods can be used to allow clients with communication difficulties to be included in decision-making and evaluation of therapy. For example Parr *et al.* (2003) used narratives to get information about the experiences, feelings and thoughts of people with aphasia concerning their communication disorder, recovery and solutions that have helped them to build up their lives again.

In the preparation of questionnaires and conduct of interviews a multimodal approach may be more effective for people with communication difficulties; that is using speech, writing, drawing and gestures simultaneously (Holland, 1998; Hirsch and Holland, 2000; Hilari and Byng, 2003). A pictorial version of a visual analogue scale for measuring mood in people with neurological conditions has been shown to be as valid as the version without pictures (Stern *et al.*, 1997). People with severe and moderate aphasia have been found to estimate their own communication skills quite similarly with their care givers when the questionnaires have been modified with pictures to be aphasia-friendly (Rautakoski *et al.*, 2008). Visual prompts have also been used successfully as augmentative means of communication in studies of psychosocial well-being and quality of life (Hoen *et al.*, 1997; Engell *et al.*, 2003). Text modifications, like simplified vocabulary and syntax, bigger font and only a few lines on a page, have also been used successfully (Brennan *et al.*, 2005). For example, Hilari and Byng (2003) used such modifications in their questionnaire, the Stroke Specific Quality of Life Scale.

Reflections on incorporating client views into SLT practice

SLTs have long known that the perspective of the client is very important in assessing the difficulty, planning the goals of the intervention and evaluating the outcomes of it. However, it is probably true to say that it is not yet routine in our work to consider the personal opinions of the client, as the principle focus is often still on the 'impairment' level. The ICF framework supports a more social model of understanding and working with clients, and this model emphasizes the importance of working collaboratively with clients and understanding their disorder within a broader social context.

Our own discipline is quite new and in many ways we are just developing our own methods and perspectives. In addition, our therapy methods are under constant development. It is important that in our own research and clinical interventions, the 'insider perspective' of the client is taken into account. In this way, we will have interventions that increasingly support the quality of life of our clients.

References

Behrmann, A. (2005) Common practices of voice therapists in the evaluation of patients. *Journal of Voice*, **19**, 454–469.

Brennan, A.D., Worrall, L.E. and McKenna, K.T. (2005) The relationship between specific features of aphasia-friendly written material for people with aphasia: An explanatory study. *Aphasiology*, **19**, 693–711.

Byng, S., Cairns, D. and Duchan, J. (2002) Values in practice and practicing values. *Journal of Communication Disorders*, **35**, 89–106.

Byng, S. and Duchan, J. (2005) Social model philosophics and principles: Their applications to therapies for aphasia. *Aphasiology*, **19**, 906–922.

Chapey, R., Duchan, J., Elman, R., *et al.* (2000) Life participation approach to aphasia: A statement of values for the future. *ASHA Leader*, **5** (3), 4–6.

Eadie, T., Yorkston, K., Klasner, E., *et al.* (2006) Measuring communicative participation: A review of self-report instruments in speech-language pathology. *American Journal of Speech-Language Pathology*, **15**, 307–320.

Engell, B., Hütter, B.-O., Willems, K. and Huber, W. (2003) Quality of life in aphasia: Validation of a pictorial self-rating procedure. *Aphasiology*, **17**, 383–396.

Franic, D.M., Bramlett, R.E. and Bothe, A.C. (2005) Psychometric evaluation of disease specific quality of life instruments in voice disorders. *Journal of Voice*, **19**, 300–315.

Hilari, K. and Byng, S. (2003) Measuring quality of life in people with aphasia: The stroke specific quality scale. *International Journal of Language and Communication Disorders*, **36**, 89–91.

Hirsch, F.M. and Holland, A.L. (2000) Beyond activity: Measuring participation in society and quality of life. In L. Worrall and C. Frattali (eds), *Neurogenic Communication Disorders: A Functional Approach*. New York: Thieme, pp. 35–54.

Hoen, B., Thelander, M. and Worsley, J. (1997) Improvement in psychological well-being of people with aphasia and their families: Evaluation of a community-based programme. *Aphasiology*, **11**, 681–691.

Hogikyan, N.D. and Sethuraman, G. (1999) Validation of an instrument to measure Voice-Related Quality of Life (V-RQOL). *Journal of Voice*, **13**, 557–569.

Holland, A. (1991) Pragmatic aspects of intervention in aphasia. *Journal of Neurolinguistics*, **6**, 197–211.

Holland, A. (1998) Functional outcome assessment of aphasia following left hemisphere stroke. *Seminars in Speech and Language*, **19**, 249–260.

Jacobson, B.H., Johnson, A., Grywalski, C., *et al.* (1997). The Voice Handicap Index (VHI): Development and validation. *American Journal of Speech-Language Pathology*, **6**, 66–70.

Kagan, A. (1998) Supported conversation for adults with aphasia: Methods and resources for training conversation partners. *Aphasiology*, **12**, 816–830.

Kagan, A. and Duchan, J. (2004) Consumers' views of what makes therapy worthwhile. In J. Duchan and S. Byng (eds), *Challenging Aphasia Therapies. Broadening the Discourse and Extending the Boundaries*. Hove, UK: Psychology Press, pp. 158–172.

Kagan, A. and Gailey, G.F. (1993). Functional is not enough. Training conversation partners for aphasic adults. In A.L. Holland and M.M. Forbes (eds), *Aphasia Treatment: World Perspectives*. San Diego: Singular.

Kagan, A., Black, E.S., Duchan, J.F., Simmons-Mackie, N. and Square, P. (2001) Training volunteers as conversation partners using 'Supported conversation for adults with aphasia' (SCA): A controlled trial. *Journal of Speech, Language and Hearing Research*, **44**, 624–638.

Krischke, S., Weigelt, S., Hoppe, U., *et al.* (2005). Quality of Life in dysphonic patients. *Journal of Voice*, **19**, 132–137.

LeDorze, G. and Brassard, C. (1995) A description of the consequences of aphasia on aphasic persons and their relatives and friends based on the WHO model of chronic diseases. *Aphasiology*, **9**, 239–255.

Lyon, J.G., Cariski, D., Keisler, L., *et al.* (1997) Communication partners: Enhancing participation in life and communication for adults with aphasia in natural settings. *Aphasiology*, **11**, 693–708.

McHorney, C.A., Robbins, J., Lomax, K., *et al.* (2002) The SWAL-QOL and SWAL-CARE outcomes tool for oropharyngeal dysphagia in adults: III. Documentation of reliability and validity. *Dysphagia*, **17**, 97–114.

Morris, J., Howard, D. and Kennedy, S. (2004) The value of therapy: What counts? In J. Duchan and S. Byng (eds), *Challenging Aphasia Therapies. Broadening the Discourse and Extending the Boundaries*. Hove, UK: Psychology Press, pp. 134–157.

Parr, S. and Byng, S. (2000) Perspectives and priorities: Accessing user views in functional communication assessment. In L. Worrall and C. Frattali (eds), *Neurogenic Communication Disorders: A Functional Approach*. New York: Thieme, pp. 55–66.

Parr, S., Duchan, J. and Pound, C. (2003) *Aphasia Inside Out: Reflections on Communication Disability*. Maidenhead, UK: Open University Press.

Pound, C., Parr, S. and Duchan, J. (2001) Using partners' autobiographical reports to develop, deliver, and evaluate services in aphasia. *Aphasiology*, **15**, 477–493.

Pound, C., Parr, S., Lindsay, J. and Woolf, C. (2002) *Beyond Aphasia. Therapies for Living with Communication Disability*. Milton Keynes, UK: Speechmark.

Ramsberger, G. (1994) Functional perspective for assessment and rehabilitation of persons with severe aphasia. *Seminars in Speech and Language*, **15**, 1–16.

Rautakoski, P., Korpijaakko-Huuhka, A.-M. and Klippi, A. (2008) People with severe and moderate aphasia and their partners as estimators of communicative skills: A client-centred evaluation. *Aphasiology*, **22**, 1269–1293.

Sarno, M.T. (1997) Quality of life in aphasia in the first post-stoke year. *Aphasiology*, **11**, 665–679.

Stern, R.A., Arruda, J.E., Hooper, C.R., Wolfner, G.D. and Morey, C.E. (1997) Visual analogue mood scales to measure internal mood state in neurologically impaired patients: Description and initial validity evidence. *Aphasiology*, **11**, 59–71.

World Health Organization (2001) *International Classification of Functioning, Disability and Health (ICF)*. Geneva: WHO.

Worrall, L. (2000) *FCTP: Functional Communication Therapy Planner*. Bicester, UK: Winslow Press.

Worrall, L. (2006) Professionalism and functional outcomes. *Journal of Communication Disorders*, **39**, 320–327.

Yaruss, J.S. (1998) Describing the consequences of disorders: Stuttering and the international classification of impairments, disabilities, and handicaps. *Journal of Speech, Language and Hearing Research*, **49**, 249–257.

Yaruss, J.S. and Quesal, R.W. (2006) Overall assessment of the Speaker's Experience of Stuttering (OASES): Documenting multiple outcomes in stuttering treatment. *Journal of Fluency Disorders*, **31**, 90–115.

16

Developing evidence-based clinical resources

Russell Thomas Cross

Vice President AAC Product Development, Prentke Romich Company, Wooster, OH, USA

As a speech and language therapist (SLT) who has worked in the field of augmentative and alternative communication (AAC) for 20 years, an on-going challenge has been to monitor how a client uses an AAC system, and to then use the results inform clinical action. Data about how clients are using an AAC device is critical for clinicians to evaluate whether or not that client is able to use it to communicate effectively. Having access to performance data like this is a key feature of evidence-based practice (EBP) (Logemann, 2000), and supports clinicians to evaluate not only the changes in behaviour of the client, but also the efficacy of the treatment itself. With current technology, there is the potential for clinicians to record all use of an augmentative communication device, which can then be used to accurately evaluate a client's current linguistic functioning. In this chapter, I will describe an approach which I developed based on the current evidence base, and which can be used to support clinicians working in the area of AAC to evaluate client communication.

Sampling communication in AAC: the problem of too much data

People with severe communication difficulties may use a speech generating device (SGD) or voice output communication aid (VOCA) with assistance from a SLT with expertise in AAC. Such technology operates by providing a client with prestored letters, words, phrases, or sentences, with either a recorded or synthetic voice. Clients access stored messages in whichever way is best for them: direct selection of a key; clicking on a switch to scan through and select items; using a head-pointing mechanism; or using an eye-gaze system. Clients with limited physical abilities or cognitive impairments may take a long time to generate even a single sentence. This makes it easy for a clinician to hand-record data but almost impossible to develop future therapy plans. However, gathering data on a daily basis provides a clinician with a much larger sample. With more data, the clinician can determine specific areas of intervention on which to focus, such as vocabulary practice, vocabulary expansion, or system use instruction (Hill and Romich, 2000).

Data collection in assistive technology is referred to as automated data logging (ADL) or language activity monitoring (LAM); both types of data collection are referred to as ADL for the rest of this chapter. The data obtained from ADL may be used as input in making best-practice decisions. Moreover, more and more studies are using ADL to evaluate intervention strategies and client improvements (for example, Higginbotham *et al.*, 1999; Tullman and Hurtubise, 2000; Cross, 2005), and research continues to establish common standards for device operation measurements. Present technology can monitor and record various types of events for clinicians to review. Different devices provide different types of data but generally the information collected includes:

- access method (such as single switch, headpointing, and direct selection)
- time
- message
- encoding method used (for example, logical letter encoding, symbols, or words).

Once data have been collected, the findings have to be processed either manually or by software. Such software includes SALT (Miller and Chapman, 1983), AQUA (Higginbotham *et al.*, 1999; Lesher *et al.*, 2000), and PERT (Romich *et al.*, 2003). Data are saved as a file that can be opened by either a specific program designed for analysing such files (e.g. ACQUA, PERT) or a common multipurpose program that can import the file (e.g. Microsoft Excel). Both types of program essentially take raw data and put it into some sort of order that a clinician can read. The clinical component of the process is to look at ordered data, make inferences about what it reveals regarding the client's use of the device, and then plan therapeutic intervention. For example, time-stamped samples allow the clinician to calculate words per minute, useful as a baseline measure followed by regular re-evaluations to track changes in communication rate. A clinician might also count the number of different words in a sample versus the total number of words and calculate a type-token ratio, a measure of lexical richness.

Although the different software programs can give detailed descriptive information about the client's language output, a key problem is that analysing the data can take some time. For most clinicians, time to perform a detailed computer-based analysis is limited. There may also be the need to pre-tag vocabulary items so that the software can actually perform an analysis. Thus, these software programs may not suit the needs of the busy SLT clinician. However, even without using such software, it is possible to use the raw data to get an overview of a client's communication skills and gain information of such issues as:

- rate of utterance
- encoding method
- vocabulary size
- morphological development.

Supporting clinicians to sort through the data: the QUAD profile

The Quick AAC Developmental Profile (QUAD Profile) is an adjunct tool to the software programs mentioned above. The goal of the QUAD Profile is to provide a tool that enables a clinician to perform a simple, rapid evaluation of the language performance of a client who is using a SGD or VOCA. Clinicians utilize the printed data generated by ADLs and compare these against a checklist focused on vocabulary, morphology, syntax, and semantics/pragmatics. The QUAD tool uses developmental norms to allow comparisons with normal language growth. By focusing on these four areas, a better overview of a client's linguistic functioning can be achieved. The QUAD assumes that the client is generating spontaneous language and not simply using lists of pre-stored whole sentences.

Evidence-based development of the QUAD

Vocabulary

The first step in developing the QUAD was to measure vocabulary use. The question being asked was, 'Is the client able to use normal vocabulary as compared with that of speaking individuals?' In short, can we match the client's vocabulary used with other vocabulary lists? To do this, a composite list was generated from several studies. These have shown that a relatively small number of words are used for most of our conversation (Howes, 1966; Hofland and Johannson, 1984; Leech et al., 2001). This is true of normally developing children (Raban, 1987), and individuals using AAC systems (Beukelman et al., 1991; Fried-Oaken and More, 1992; Marvin et al., 1994; Stuart et al., 1997).

Using Microsoft Excel a vocabulary set was created of words that appeared (a) across ages, (b) across client groups, and (c) were high frequency. For example, words such as I, want, that and have will be found in words lists of children and adults. This list provided the basis for a generic core set of 260 words that could be used as a checklist to match against an ADL file.

An important point to note is that the QUAD list is 'noun poor' because these are actually the most variable group across vocabulary studies. Nouns change across time, ages, and groups, and also have very low frequencies of use. The word dog may certainly be used by a five-year-old and its inclusion in an AAC system may be valuable, but adding it to a generic high frequency list makes little sense. QUAD explicitly avoids these.

Morphology

The next stage in the design of the QUAD was to ask the question, 'Does the client show evidence of using normal developmental morphology?' The ability to use morphology is a critical component of not just the English language (Blockberger and Johnston, 2003; Tomasello, 2006; Waxman and Lidz, 2005) but all languages (Pinker, 1999; Deutscher, 2005). Brown (1973) outlined a developmental sequence for the acquisition of morphology in the English language and this has been used extensively as a benchmark by clinicians. Brown's morphemes have been used in a number of analytical tools such as the LARSP (Crystal *et al.*, 1976), and SALT (Miller and Chapman, 1983).

Syntax

The third question asked was, 'Does the client show the ability to generate sentences based on the normal rules of English grammar?' From a very early age, children are able to learn that words can be categorized as parts of speech (Waxman and Gelman, 1986), and even use these categories to attach meaning to words (Hall and Lavin, 2004). Adults frequently add new words to their mental dictionary and can typically use all the correct forms of the word once they know its grammatical category (Prasada and Pinker, 1993; Dabrowska, 2004). The rules that describe how parts of speech can vary are well documented (Huddleston and Pullum, 2005; Quirk and Greenbaum, 1990) and using these rules in any language system is recommended. Specifically, the QUAD drew heavily from the LARSP model and includes a checklist of the basic sentence types.

Semantics/pragmatics

The final question asked was, 'How does the client appear to be using language?' For simplicity, the seven-point classification used by Halliday (1975) was used. As there are only a limited number of choices, and each is fairly wide in terms of description, the clinician does not need to spend a lot of time with the analysis – the aim is to provide a 'broad brush' overview. The functions of language that are sampled using the QUAD are shown in Figure 16.1.

Using the QUAD: a clinical example

Amber is a 22-year-old woman diagnosed with an atypical degenerative ataxic syndrome at 18 years of age. She had been using an SGD since August 2005 with a word-based language application called WordCore (Cross, 2004; Cross and Tullman, 2006). Access to the device is via two switches placed at each side of her head. A number of separate data samples were collected over a two-week period, each one a different length. After a short period of automated data collection, a QUAD analysis was performed and the following simple observations made.

- *Vocabulary.* The sample from Amber contained 66 of the 237 core words in the QUAD profile, representing 28% of the set. Examples of these high frequency core words included *I*, *the*, *to*, *and*, *you*, *it* and *did*. Using so many core words is a positive indicator because core words account for some 80% of all vocabulary used (Vanderheiden and Kelso, 1987).
- *Morphology.* Amber used examples of 12 of the possible 16 morphemes in the QUAD Morphology Checklist. An important aspect of the QUAD is that the checklist can also be used to drive further investigation. For example, with this client it was possible to set up clinical scenarios designed to elicit the missing forms. The QUAD is not a normative test but a snap-shot overview, and as such, it is perfectly legitimate to use it to 'teach to test' – using the QUAD feedback to modify the client's behavior.

Enter a date for a week/month and simply check off, in the column below, instances where each sentence type is observed.

Age	Type	Example	Date	Date	Date	Date	Date
9–12 months	Instrumental	requesting things asking for physical help quantifier ("more") "I want ... "					
9–12 months	Regulatory	"Do as I say" controlling others					
9–12 months	Interactional	information exchange "me and you" statements greetings and social					
9–12 months	Personal	maintaining contact interests "I feel ... "					
16–35 months	Heuristic	asserting identity "tell me why" discovery choices					
16–35 months	Imaginative	let's pretend creative imagery					
16–35 months	Informative	statements of fact story telling					

Figure 16.1 QUAD Checklist for language functions (semantics/pragmatics).

- *Syntax.* Amber was able to create complex sentence types that included such devices as coordination ('Sorry I can't be there but it is not wheelchair accessible') and ellipsis ('Yes I did get the last one you sent me'.) Error sentences included 'It's really frustrating when I am talking to somebody and they can't understand me'. By looking briefly at the data and comparing it to the QUAD's syntax section it became clear that she has a good command of English and was very aware of 'correct' grammar. She was clearly able to use the device effectively to create these complex sentences – an important observation for planning future therapy.
- *Semantic/pragmatics.* Sentences such as the one beginning 'It's really is frustrating ...' illustrate what Halliday (1975) calls the' Personal function' – comments about feelings and interests. Other example sentences include 'How about yourself?' (the Interactional function); 'I am using a device to write e-mails' (Informative function); 'Did you download that book?' (Heuristic function); and 'Stephen King horror stories carry jokes' (Imaginative function). It isn't critical that every sentence is analysed in great detail because the check-

list is designed to serve as a guideline as to what function to look for. If a client provides evidence of using all seven types of function that is a positive result; if only a few forms are used, that suggests further investigation is needed.

Reflections on developing an evidence-based tool

Trying to design a tool that was easy to use yet that provided useful data took me many months and it represents a working clinician's tool rather than a researcher's test. A major challenge in creating the QUAD was in balancing simplicity against validity. It became a 'profile' because it was never intended to be a rigorous, normative tool with standardized measures but a simple clinical tool that highlights areas of concern. The age ranges included are merely guidelines, not prescriptions. Some clinicians have criticized the QUAD precisely because it is not standardized. However, others have been simply happy to have it as a means of helping them focus on how to analyse their data.

Clinicians who work in the area of AAC are often faced with the challenge of evaluating two things: the client's communicative abilities, and their ability to use the AAC device (SGA or VOCA) optimally. The QUAD tool is a simple method to support clinicians to evaluate clients and to support clinical decision-making. Its design has been based on the best available evidence about vocabulary, syntax and morphology development is intended to guide therapy, and hence support reflective, EBP.

References

Beukelman, D.R., McGinnis, J. and Morrow, D. (1991) Vocabulary selection in augmentative and alternative communication. *Augmentative and Alternative Communication*, 7, 171–185.

Blockberger, S. and Johnston, J. (2003) Grammatical morphology acquisition by children with complex communication needs. *Augmentative and Alternative Communication*, **19**, 207–221.

Brown, R. (1973) *A First Language: The Early Stages*. Cambridge, MA: Harvard University Press.

Cross, R.T. (2004) WordCore© 84: Communication Software For The Vantage/Vanguard Communication Aids. Proceedings of the International Society for Augmentative and Alternative Communication Biennial Conference, Natal, (pp. 304–306). Toronto: ISAAC.

Cross, R.T. (2005) Language activity monitoring: profiling and planning therapy. Paper presented at the American Speech–Language–Hearing Association Conference, San Diego.

Cross, R.T. and Tullman, J. (2006) WordCore© 84 AAC communication program: updates and a case study. Proceedings of the International Society for Augmentative and Alternative Communication Biennial Conference, Duesseldorf, (pp. 613–614). Toronto: ISAAC.

Crystal, D., Fletcher, P. and Garman, M. (1976) *The Grammatical Analysis of Language Disability*. London: Arnold.

Dabrowska, E. (2004) Rules or schemas? Evidence from Polish. *Language and Cognitive Processes*, **19**, 225–271.

Deutscher, G. (2005) *The Unfolding of Language: An Evolutionary Tour of Mankind's Greatest Invention*. London: William Heinemann.

Fried-Oaken, M. and More, L. (1992) An initial vocabulary for nonspeaking preschool children based on developmental and environmental language sources. *Augmentative and Alternative Communication*, 8, 41–54.

Hall, D.G. and Lavin, T.A. (2004) The use and misuse of part-of-speech information in word learning: Implications for lexical development. In D.G. Hall and S.R. Waxman (eds), *Weaving a Lexicon*. Cambridge, MA: MIT Press.

Halliday, M.A.K. (1975) *Learning how to Mean*. London: Edward Arnold.

Higginbotham, D.J., Lesher, G.W. and Moulton, B.J. (1999) Development of a voluntary format for augmentative communication device log files. Proceedings of the 1999 Rehabilitation Engineering and Assistive Technology Society of North America (RESNA) (pp. 25–27). Arlington, VA: RESNA Press.

Hill, K. and Romich, B. (2000) AAC best practice using automated language activity monitoring. Proceedings of the International Society for Augmentative and Alternative Communication Biennial Conference, (pp. 761–764). Toronto: ISAAC.

Hofland, S. and Johannson, K. (1984) *Word Frequencies in British and American English*. Bergen: Longman.

Howes, D. (1966) A word count of spoken English. *Journal of Verbal Learning and Verbal Behavior*, **5**, 572–604.

Huddleston, R. and Pullum, G.K. (2005) *A Student's Introduction to English Grammar*. Cambridge: Cambridge University Press.

Leech, G., Rayson, P. and Wilson, A. (2001) *Word Frequencies in Written and Spoken English, Based on the British National Corpus*. London: Longman.

Lesher, G.W., Moulton, B.J., Rinkus, G. and Higginbotham, D.J. (2000) A universal logging format for augmentative communication. Proceedings of the Annual International Conference on Technology and Persons with Disabilities (CSUN). Retrieved 8 October 2009 from http://www.csun.edu/cod/conf/2000/proceedings/0088Lesher.htm

Logemann, J. (2000) What is evidence-based practice and why should we care? *ASHA Leader*, 5 (5), 3.

Marvin, C.A., Beukelman, D.R. and Bilyeu, D. (1994) Vocabulary use patterns in preschool children: effects of context and time sampling. *Augmentative and Alternative Communication*, **10**, 224–236.

Miller, J.F. and Chapman, R.S. (1983) *Systematic Analysis of Language Transcripts (SALT)*. San Diego: College Hills Press.

Pinker, S. (1999) *Words and Rules: The Ingredients of Language*. New York: Basic Books.

Prasada, S. and Pinker, S. (1993) Generalisations of regular and irregular morphological patterns. *Language and Cognitive Processes*, 8, 1–56.

Quirk, R. and Greenbaum, S. (1990) *A Student's Grammar of the English Language*. Harlow, UK: Longman.

Raban, B. (1987) *The Spoken Vocabulary of Five-Year-Old Children*. Reading, UK: The Reading and Language Information Centre.

Romich, B.A., Hill, K., Seagull, A., Ahmad, N., Strecker, J. and Gotla, K. (2003) AAC performance report tool: PERT. Proceedings of the Rehabilitation Engineering and Assistive Technology Society of North America (RESNA) Annual Conference, RESNA Press.

Stuart, S., Beukelman, D.R. and King, J. (1997) Vocabulary use during extended conversations by two cohorts of older adults. *Augmentative and Alternative Communication*, **13**, 40–47.

Tomasello, M. (2006) Acquiring linguistic constructions. In D. Kuhn and R. Siegler (eds), *Handbook of Child Psychology*. New York: Wiley, pp. 255–298.

Tullman, J. and Hurtubise, C. (2000) Language activity monitoring on a young child using a VOCA. Proceedings of the International Society for Augmentative and Alternative Communication Biennial Conference Proceedings, Washington, (pp. 300–313). Toronto: ISSAC.

Vanderheiden, G.C. and Kelso, D.P. (1987) Comparative analysis of fixed-vocabulary communication acceleration techniques. *Augmentative and Alternative Communication*, **3**, 196–206.

Waxman, S.R. and Gelman, R. (1986) Preschoolers' use of superordinate relations in classification and language. *Cognitive Development*, **1** (2), 139–156.

Waxman, S.R. and Lidz, J.L. (2005). Early word learning. In D. Kuhn and R. Siegler (eds), *Handbook of Child Psychology*. New York: Wiley.

17

Creating evidence-based policy to facilitate evidence-based practice

Angie Dobbrick

Senior Speech Pathologist, Royal Brisbane and Women's Hospital,
Brisbane, Australia

The Royal Brisbane and Women's Hospital (RBWH) is part of Queensland Health (QH). It is currently a 982 bed, tertiary referral teaching hospital with a number of specialties. It is the largest tertiary referral hospital in Queensland and provides services to patients throughout the State, northern New South Wales, the Northern Territory and from neighbouring countries in the south-west Pacific. The speech and language therapy (SLT) department is one of many allied health departments that services the hospital. It is a reasonably large department of approximately 18 full time positions and more than 20 staff. As part of my Senior role I am responsible for staff and delivery of services in medicine both acute and post acute.

QH has an emphasis on the development of evidence-based policies to guide hospital practices. With this in mind each SLT staff member, regardless of years of experience or position in the department, is encouraged to carry out quality improvement (QI) projects. Some of these may involve the development of policies, either at a hospital or department level. Staff are supported to undertake these projects, and may be eligible for RBWH or QH grant/funding opportunities to assist and support us in carrying these projects out. This chapter outlines a particular QI project, focusing on the development and implementation of the Royal Brisbane Dysphagia Screening Tool (DST) and its supporting policies. This example shows how implementing evidence-based policy can facilitate evidence-based practice (EBP). The majority of the development of the DST was undertaken prior to my working at the RBWH. However, when I was appointed as Senior Speech and Language Therapist at the RBWH my responsibilities regarding the DST included mentoring staff, attending meetings, and its rollout.

Background to the RBWH Dysphagia Screening Tool and policy

Historically, patients admitted to RBWH were not routinely screened for dysphagia, even if their diagnosis (e.g. stroke) put them at high risk for swallowing difficulties. Clinical staff referred for SLT assessment sporadically, meaning that some patients were at high risk of aspiration, without ever being referred for assessment by speech and language therapists. The RBWH DST was developed with the aim to enable earlier identification and management of patients with dysphagia/aspiration risk. It was designed to be performed as part of an initial admission nursing 'risk screening' assessment, to be used on all patients who fitted the 'at risk' category. Therefore, all staff needed to be made alert to dysphagia risks so that they could refer appropriately.

Given the implications of the DST for clinical practice across the hospital, a hospital-wide policy for dysphagia screening was necessary. The policy was developed alongside the screening tool to provide clear evidence for why the assessment was being carried out, and to provide staff with some infrastructure for why and how it is to be used, and the training required to use it. Without the policy to support it the DST would be likely to be used incorrectly, in an *ad hoc* manner, or not used at all. Having a fully endorsed hospital policy ensured that training and compliance were made compulsory at RBWH. Thus, the policy enabled the implementation of dysphagia screening EBP, using the DST, across the hospital.

Developing evidence-based policy

Identifying the problem and getting organizational support

In the case of the DST, a clinical incident brought dysphagia screening to our attention. We have an incident reporting system (PRIME) that is available to all clinical staff to report any incidents that may have occurred. These are then reviewed by our Safety and Quality Unit and if required forwarded on to the relevant staff/departments for further action. As part of this a risk analysis is carried out, which in this case identified a very high risk at an organizational level. A review of this case and the risk analysis showed that a hospital-wide approach was needed for dysphagia screening. It was evident that we needed to investigate the evidence to find the best approach for dysphagia screening, so as to ensure that patients were identified and managed appropriately. Identifying this issue and rating its risk gave direction to the project and made goal setting much easier. It also helped to define what evidence we were looking for and what to rule out.

Having identified such a high risk to the organization helped our case for the urgency of change in relation to dysphagia management. There was a strong possibility of negative outcomes for patients, and the spectre of litigation in the future for the hospital managers to consider. Thus, the organizational risk identified through the incident management and response process was the key in gaining support to move forward with strategies to resolve the issue. Other data supporting the process of identifying the problem and gaining support may include chart audits, and/ or analysis of organizational data, and these can be used strategically to raise the issue at appropriate forums within the service.

Gathering the evidence

Once we'd identified the problem and the level of risk it carried within the organization it was then important to gather evidence that would help inform system and policy changes with regards to dysphagia screening. This evidence also helped us in writing a business case that funded a research assistant to carry out some of the DST development and policy writing. This certainly took the burden off clinicians trying to do it in their own time.

A complete review of the literature was carried out. We examined the evidence for:

- clinical risk factors that could be used as indicators for identifying someone who may be at risk for dysphagia/aspiration
- screening for dysphagia, including existing screening tools and their psychometric properties (validity, reliability)
- the administration of screening tools or identification of clinical risk factors by different health professionals (e.g. nurses, other clinical staff)
- training, and the impact on reliability in administration of dysphagia screening tools.

Across all of these areas, the evidence base for the development of the DST policy was guided by three pertinent questions.

- How relevant is this evidence to what we are seeking to decide?
- How representative is it of our population?
- How reliable and well founded is this theoretically and empirically?

Our starting place for seeking evidence was in published empirical research. We found it useful to use a broad search that included seeking evidence outside the profession's evidence base, such as nursing journals. Additionally, we examined local and national recommendations and guidelines. For example the National Stroke Foundation's guidelines for clinical practice state that all stroke patients should be screened for dysphagia within 24 hours (National Stroke Foundation Australia, 2007). These evidence-based guidelines were taken into consideration, as were position papers from Speech Pathology Australia (Speech Pathology Australia, 2004).

Another aspect that was very important for us when gathering evidence was benchmarking. Lenz *et al.* (1994) state the benchmarking is useful in 'comparing practices and processes to identify and actualize opportunities.' We carried out our benchmarking for dysphagia screening practices in hospitals within Queensland, interstate, and internationally. It was done by developing and asking a 'loose' set of questions that were felt to be relevant in informing the project. For example: What is the difference between screening and assessment? Who can carry out dysphagia screening? What evidence is there at screening is valid and reliable? Carrying out the benchmarking, particularly the practices of other facilities with regard to dysphagia screening, helped us to gain practical knowledge from clinicians and managers. These people wrestle with everyday problems of effectiveness and implementation and collecting this knowledge not only helped to facilitate networking but also helped us in understanding how things can be most effectively implemented. It also gave us a chance to learn from other's mistakes and to see that at times we didn't have to 'reinvent the wheel' entirely. In fact, we initially hoped that this exercise might identify a model of dysphagia management which could be implemented in RBWH, or modified to suit our needs. However, as we were unable to identify something entirely suitable, we proceeded with the development of our own DST.

Local data were also important to informing our direction in relation to dysphagia management at RBWH. We examined clinical information such as length of stay, and morbidity and mortality of particular diagnosis categories. This data helped us to see what is happening at a local level and enabled us to compare this with our benchmarking and literature review results. We also examined organizational goals, business plans and any other professional policies. This was key, as we needed to ensure that our direction with the DST was compatible with existing policies and procedures within the hospital (Speech Pathology Australia, 2004; National Stroke Foundation Australia, 2007).

Our evidence review and data gathering suggested that initial identification of patients at risk of dysphagia could be undertaken by nursing staff based on indicators of clinical risk: for example, stroke, bulbar signs. However, existing tools to facilitate this identification were not suitable, and one would need to be created.

Consultation

Once the literature review, analysis of data and benchmarking were carried out we began some initial rounds of consultation to ensure anything that we might propose would be feasible and endorsed by stakeholders. Consultation was one of the most important steps to our policy development. This process supported our understanding of organizational and issue histories, and was crucial for gaining support for what we were trying to achieve.

For our purpose, consultation was approached formally. A steering group was set up called the Swallowing Assessment and Feeding Risk working group. The role of this multidisciplinary working group was 'to develop policy, strategies and actions to manage the risk associated with swallowing and feeding disorders' for the hospital (The Royal Brisbane and Women's Hospital, 2002). The membership of this steering group included a member of the hospital Executive Management group, nursing representatives from various departments, dieticians, representatives from hotel services (who provide the hospital meals), and medical staff. This group reported to two committees – the Clinical Services Committee, and Executive Committee. The inclusion of a member of the hospital Executive on our steering group was useful for garnering support and endorsement for any recommendations at the highest level. It was important to ensure all issues, purpose and directions were understood and supported by all stakeholders. The processes of governance – accountabilities, roles, decision making, resourcing, and reporting also needed to be well defined and agreed upon from the outset, along with agreement and understanding of short-, medium- and long-term goals to be achieved. From the outset, we aimed for agreement within the steering group that the policy to be developed would be a long-term, sustainable policy, and not a 'quick fix' or short-term project. We knew that if this wasn't agreed upon and supported, achieving EBP in relation to dysphagia management across the hospital would not be sustained.

The role of the steering group varied throughout the project. We used members to gain feedback about the DST as versions of the tool and policy were developed. The steering group also facilitated discussion and problem solving around implementation, for example the practicality of administering the DST when patients were admitted to RBWH. Training guidelines and maintenance of credentialing needed to also be negotiated, as did agreement on the contents of the policy.

The steering group was the main forum for consultation; however, we also conducted wider consultations at other forums where appropriate, to gain support or to discuss specific issues with other staff. For example, as the DST and policy were developed, it became evident that there would be workload issues and training needs for nursing staff, who would carry out the DST as part of an overall patient risk assessment. Therefore, it was very important to involve nursing staff in the consultation process. As part of the ongoing process of consultation, outside of the formalized steering group meetings, we found that we met with different stakeholders at varying frequency and lengths and at different parts of the process while the solutions were evolving.

Trial and evaluation

Several wards were specifically targeted to trial the DST with the intent to examine the validity of the tool, and to pilot processes that went alongside the policy. Specifically:

- all nursing staff on those wards were trained and credentialled to use the DST by a speech and language therapist
- patients deemed as 'at risk' based on clinical signs/indications were screened on admission to the ward
- patients who met the criteria for risk of aspiration using the screening tool, were referred to the SLT department for further assessment/management.

Throughout this trial period, feedback was sought from all of the relevant stakeholders, particularly nursing staff, and this led to some modifications to the processes. For example, feedback suggested that training was difficult to achieve for all nurses, due to the fact that some nurses routinely worked during the night and could not attend the training held during the day. This had potential implications for patients admitted after hours. This feedback resulted in another project to develop on-line training that is now available for nurses to complete in their own time. Once the trial period was finished, compliance data, timeliness and appropriateness of referrals and feedback were reviewed and minor changes to the policy were finalized. A report was tabled at the steering committee. We found that referrals were more timely and accurate, with increased identification of patients at risk of aspiration and dysphagia. With a couple of modifications the DST policy and tool was endorsed in principle by the steering committee and was then distributed by the Safety and Quality officers for broader hospital consultation and agreement. Once agreement was reached the policy was authorized by hospital management, and published.

The implementation of the policy was carried out in a staged approach once the trial period was finished. Rolling this policy out and the training involved to a hospital of over 900 beds would have been near impossible to be done all at once. Any sort of quality control of the new processes would also have been impossible to monitor. Instead, wards that were identified as having the most number of 'at risk' admissions were targeted first (e.g. the stroke unit). This allowed us to ensure that the policy was being carried out accurately and the DST was being used appropriately in one ward before moving on to the next.

Reflections

The development of an evidence-based policy for dysphagia screening at RBWH has definitely promoted evidence-based patient care, reduced length of stay and streamlined clinical referral processes. It has also facilitated research within the department, and the DST has now been validated and assessed for reliability in an acute hospital setting (Cichero *et al.*, 2009). Further, the DST and the processes that we have implemented are being considered state-wide, so that Queensland Health will be able to meet National Stroke Foundation Guidelines of dysphagia screening/assessment being performed within 24 hours of admission.

It is worth knowing, though, that this has taken two years from inception of the DST and its policy, to implementation and we are still discussing changes and reviewing the policy as part of the quality cycle. It wasn't always an easy task as the RBWH is a large institution with a complex matrix of systems and processes. Currently, we are still providing some training to the wards and carrying out chart audits to ensure the policy is still being followed and the tool still carried out in the appropriate manner. We have found that the on-line training and credentialling for the nursing staff has been received positively and is being used regularly. It seems that it is more convenient and time efficient than the face-to-face training that we initially planned. The DST and its policy are still agenda items on our staff meeting minutes, ensuring that the speech and language therapy staff regularly discuss the processes and outcomes of this policy, and raise any issues that require follow up.

The application of research and evidence in clinical practice on an every day basis can be difficult with many time and resource demands on the clinician. However, if there are good evidence-based policies and systems in place to facilitate EBP this takes the burden off the individual clinician and outcomes such as those that we have been able to achieve are possible. A hospital policy that is based on evidence, such as the DST policy that we developed, goes a long way to ensuring that EBP is implemented. A policy is enforceable, and creates an environment in which staff are expected to follow the processes outlined. This ensures a co-ordinated approach to complex problems, such as dysphagia screening/risk management in the acute setting. Creating and implementing evidence-based policies is only possible with careful planning, gathering of evidence, consultation, and organizational support.

References

Cichero, J.A.Y., Heaton, S.G., Bassett, L. and Lincoln, D. (2009) Triaging dysphagia: Nurse screening for dysphagia in an acute hospital. *Journal of Clinical Nursing*, **18** (11), 1649–1659.

Lenz, M., Myers, S., Nordlund, S., Sullivan, D. and Vasista, V. (1994) Benchmarking: finding ways to improve. *Joint Commission Journal on Quality Improvement*, 20 (5), 250–259.

National Stroke Foundation Australia (2007) Guidelines. Retrieved 8 October 2009 from http://www.strokefoundation.com.au/clinical-guidelines

Speech Pathology Australia (2004) Dysphagia general position paper. Melbourne: SPA.

The Royal Brisbane and Women's Hospital (2002) Terms of Reference for the Swallowing Assessment and Feeding Risk Working Group. Brisbane: RBWH.

18 Building and supporting a multi-stream clinical evidence-based practice Network

Tracy Kelly[1], Rachel Miles Kingma[2] and
Rachelle Robinson[1]

[1]*Speech Pathologist, Prince of Wales Hospital, NSW, Australia*
[2]*Speech Pathologist, War Memorial Hospital Waverley, NSW, Australia*

It is generally agreed that speech and language therapists (SLTs) should be using evidence-based practice (EBP) to support their clinical management of communication and swallowing disorders. However, the task of implementing EBP into everyday practice can be challenging. SLTs face many barriers in implementing EBP, particularly lack of time, training, and potentially limited access to resources (Quinn *et al.*, 2002; Vallino-Napoli and Reilly, 2004).

New South Wales has a population of approximately 6.7 million, living in an area of around 800 000 km², distributed across four contrasting regions: major cities (71.4%), inner regional areas (20.6%), outer regional areas (7.3%) and remote/very remote areas (0.7%) (Australian Bureau of Statistics, 2008). Responsibility for healthcare is shared between the federal and state governments, involving both public and private sectors. The New South Wales (NSW) Speech Pathology EBP Network was established in 2002 to share the task of EBP in a collaborative forum. The Network was instigated by several senior NSW Health SLT's working in acute teaching hospitals. The Network's primary objective has been to support SLTs to share the task of identifying, critically appraising and applying the evidence, and to encourage joint learning across clinicians (Quinn *et al.*, 2002).

The Network has aimed to link practising SLTs from across the state of NSW into clinically based groups, in order for clinicians working in the same fields to undertake efficient and effective review and application of the available clinical evidence. Clinicians are able to access a central web site, which details the current clinical groups. If they are interested in participating in appraising evidence in these topic areas, they can contact the group leader, and attend training. Groups choose the topics for appraisal, and work together on this task. They produce both critically appraised topics (CATs) and critically appraised papers (CAPs). A CAP is an easily digested summary of a critical review of a research paper, in response to the clinical question. A CAT is the overall summary of the critical review of all the best available evidence on a particular topic – a collation of all the CAPs. Both documents are written outcomes of the EBP process and provide useful summaries for clinicians to use in practice.

This chapter will outline the structure and processes of the NSW EBP Network, as well as concluding with a discussion of issues surrounding establish and maintenance of such a Network.

Framework of the Network

The general framework of the EBP Network is outlined in Figure 18.1. The NSW Speech Pathology EBP Network is coordinated by a steering committee of three members as a voluntary adjunct to their full time clinical and/or managerial speech pathology roles in NSW Health.

The Steering Committee (SC) is responsible for coordination of all EBP Network activities. The SC provides the training for clinicians who wish to join the EBP Network and provides support to the clinical group leaders. The SC is also responsible for ensuring that all groups maintain a consistent approach to critical appraisal throughout the Network. The use of standard forms for reporting CATs and CAPs ensures that each group approaches these systematically. The SC coordinate the annual Network Extravaganza, where CATs and CAPs developed throughout the year are presented. They also maintain and revise the web site, which is a central point of communication for the Network.

In 2008 there were 10 clinical groups in the EBP Network:

- Adult Speech
- Adult Swallowing
- Adult Language
- Adult Tracheostomy & Critical Care
- Paediatric Phonology
- Paediatric Language
- Paediatric Feeding – Acute
- Paediatric Feeding – Disability
- Cleft Palate
- Alternative and Augmentative Communication (AAC).

Each group has between one and three leaders and ranges in size from 5 to 30 members. Leaders and members work across the state in acute and rehabilitation hospitals, community health, education and disability, in metropolitan and rural

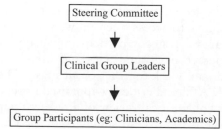

Figure 18.1 Framework of the NSW Speech Pathology EBP Network.

work settings. With such a diverse number of groups and clinicians, each group functions individually within the guidelines provided by the Network. Groups meet four to six times annually and remain in contact via e-mail between meetings. Each of the clinical groups functions differently, and each group's structure has evolved over the years, according to the members' needs and the clinical climate. Some groups meet prior to a professional development session; some are linked with a relevant clinical 'discussion' or 'interest' group; some exist independently and function entirely as an EBP group.

Clinical members are required to actively participate in the functioning of the group. This may involve formulating a clinical question; conducting literature searches; critically evaluating relevant research articles; and electronically completing CAP and CAT forms. Currently, membership is restricted to qualified SLTs working in NSW. Once clinicians have joined the Network by contacting the leader of the group that they are interested in, they must undertake training by attending a workshop on EBP (see Box 18.1). While it is acknowledged that many participants will have already undertaken some form of research methods training, this approach aims to ensure a consistency of approach across groups and an understanding of the fundamentals of the Network.

The SC conduct up to four EBP Network workshops per year. Training (a 2.5 hour workshop) has been conducted face-to-face with clinicians or via teleconferencing, or as a self-study training package. We were very sure that we did not want this training to be seen as a professional development event where people passively listen to the workshop with no further involvement once it has finished. The workshop requires prereading material, active participation during the session and an expectation that participants will join the Network by becoming an active member of a clinical group of their choice.

Leaders are responsible for ensuring that all group members participate in training and contribute to group activity. They also evaluate all CAPs and CATs created by the group prior to sending to the SC for placement on the web site. The leaders also have a number of administrative roles, such as providing feedback from their group to the SC, disseminating information from the SC to members, and maintaining a central database of members and their group's activities.

Feedback from group leaders and members suggested that interpreting data and evaluating research methodology were often challenges for members. Following discussion with clinical group leaders, those groups who reported least difficulty with these areas were those that had university academics amongst their

---

Box 18.1   Outline of the EBP Network training workshops

- Introduction to the NSW Speech Pathology EBP Network
- Principles of EBP: What is EBP?
- Formulating a clinical question
- Searching databases
- Critical appraisal of research
- Practical session: creating a critically appraised paper
- Joining the Network

membership. For this reason the SC approached various academics from all relevant universities across NSW, and invited them to join the Network. The outcome of this has been very positive, with the majority of clinical groups now having at least one academic member.

Function of the clinical groups

CAT and CAP topic areas are raised by clinicians, in line with the focus of the group. With much discussion among group members, this is then shaped into a clinical question. The importance of creating a clinical question that is relevant and answerable is an integral part of the process. Having members decide on the clinical question provides ownership and creates a vested interest, which in turn leads to greater outcomes. The EBP Network suggests that clinicians use the PICO model (patient/problem, intervention, comparison (optional) and outcomes) to formulate the clinical question (e.g. 'In tracheostomy patients, is the modified Evans Blue Dye Test effective in detecting aspiration?').

Between group meetings, members conduct a number of searches of various databases and create a list of relevant articles that answer the clinical question. These articles are then collated and critically appraised using standardized forms in order to create CAPs and CATs (see Figure 18.2). For both CAPs and CATs, clinicians create a statement about the 'clinical bottom line', which summarizes the implications of the findings. This clinical bottom line is based on the level of evidence reviewed and is formed through discussion among the group. The instructions for completing the CAT and CAP forms state that 'the clinical bottom line should be aimed to help clinicians apply what evidence there is' in a particular area. For reliability, the articles are critically appraised by at least two clinicians, and reviewed by a third clinician and/or the group leader if discrepancies exist.

To comply with the current terms of reference that were agreed upon by all clinical leaders, one CAT must be produced per year in order for a group to remain part of the Network. In 2007, all groups fulfilled this requirement, with groups completing between one and six CATs. CATs are presented at the annual Extravaganza, which is a forum to showcase the work each clinical group has produced throughout the year.

Communication processes

Web site

In order to share the information of the Network initially, the Steering Committee produced a newsletter. As the Network became more extensive a web page was created which subsequently has developed into a web site, with the support of NSW Health CIAP (Clinical Information Access Project – a web site of clinical information and resources that is designed to support EBP at the point of care). CIAP is a resource is available to all nurses, midwives, doctors, allied health, community health, ancillary and library staff working in the NSW public health system. The web site contains general information about the Network, contact

NSW Speech Pathology
Evidence Based Practice Interest Group

╔══════════════════════════════════════╗
║   **Critically Appraised Paper (CAP)**   ║
╚══════════════════════════════════════╝

CLINICAL BOTTOM LINE:

Clinical Question [patient/problem, intervention, (comparison), outcome]:

Citation:

Design/Method:

Participants:

Experimental Group:

Control Group:

Results:

Comments – Strengths/weaknesses of paper

Level of Evidence (NH&MRC):

Appraised By:
Clinical Group:

Date:

Figure 18.2 Critically appraised topic (CAT) and critically appraised paper (CAP) forms used by the NSW EBP Network. From Quinn *et al.*, 2002. Reproduced by permission of the authors. CAP form developed based on suggestions by Worrall and Bennett (2001).

NSW Speech Pathology
Evidence Based Practice Interest Group

Critically Appraised Topic (CAT)

CLINICAL BOTTOM LINE:

Background and Objectives:

Clinical Question [patient/problem, intervention, (comparison), outcome]:

Search Terms/Systems:

Selection Criteria:

Results:

Appraised By:
Clinical Group:

Date:

Figure 18.2 *Continued*

information, clinical groups, current clinical questions, completed CAPs and CATs, and up-coming workshops and education sessions. The web site is accessible to members of the NSW Speech Pathology EBP Network and also the general public, (www.ciap.health.nsw.gov.au/specialties/ebp_sp_path)

Annual EBP 'Extravaganza'

Every year, the work of each clinical group is showcased at a conference-style 'EBP Network Extravaganza'. This provides groups with an achievable goal to present the year's CATs, and the impact these summaries of evidence have made on clinical practice, to a forum of over 200 people including members, other practicing SLTs and academics. The Extravaganza has provided a forum to share information, promoted enthusiasm towards EBP, and subsequently increased active involvement in the Network. It has been particularly beneficial in reaching a larger audience of clinicians in rural areas of NSW with involvement of over 100 people via videoteleconference.

Key features of this initiative

The impact of group size

The number and size of clinical groups has changed over time with groups forming and dispersing as current clinical trends change. For example, initially there was one clinical group for clinicians focusing on adult acquired speech, swallowing and communication difficulties. While this was understandably one of the largest and most popular clinical groups, it had challenges maintaining focus due to the diverse scope of clinical practice. After a strategic planning meeting, initiated by the group leaders and facilitated by the SC, it was collaboratively agreed to split into three different clinical groups (Adult Speech; Adult Swallowing, Adult Language). While group numbers are smaller, group leaders and members report more productivity and that the groups review clinical questions that are more relevant to individual clinicians. Group members reported that this has provided more opportunities for focused discussion and learning, and increased output and quality has been noted in terms of completed CAPs and CATs.

Development of the groups from special interest/discussion groups

Initially some of the clinical groups were newly formed while others attempted to add an EBP component to their existing 'interest' or 'discussion' group. This was met with varying results with some groups flourishing by taking the opportunity to refocus their group of already dedicated clinicians into discussing clinical questions, critiquing relevant research, creating CAPs and CATs and applying EBP into clinical practice. Other established groups found resistance to changing current group structures and dynamics and EBP principles were not embraced. The difference between an EBP clinical group and a Specialist Interest Group seems to be that interest groups are often education and/or discussion based, whilst an EBP Network group is focused on creating questions, critiquing the research, producing CAPs/CATs, and discussing the application of the clinical bottom line.

Being 'clinician led'

The Network's perceived success may be based on the philosophy of the Network being clinician led. While managers initially established the Network, and there is continued strong direct support through management, the groups of clinicians are directing their own learning by being actively involved in their clinical area of interest. Clinicians join groups they are specifically interested in and as members, they develop clinical questions that will directly impact on their daily interventions, policies and procedures, and the development of guidelines.

Involvement of academics

Having academics as group members has assisted in shaping clinical questions that are answerable through these members having such extensive knowledge of current literature and research available. The academics report a great satisfaction in being part of the clinical groups of the Network alongside practising clinicians who have an interest in their specialist field. Following increased participation by academics, Network members express greater confidence in their ability to critique research also in applying the evidence. This has also facilitated stronger links with the universities and academics, and helped develop a collegial working relationship between universities, academics and clinicians.

Importance of training

The fact that all members must attend the training has supported the consistency of approach across the Network. Critiquing speech pathology research is very complex. The workshops that we provide include a general overview about these concepts. Members have also requested more in-depth knowledge and training in certain areas of EBP. Additional training workshops have been coordinated by the steering committee, in such areas as single case design, database usage, and critiquing methods. Feedback from leaders and members have led to the planning of a more advanced workshop to further extend skills of critiquing, searching and applying the evidence.

Support for clinical leaders

Support for the clinical leaders is imperative. The administration and organizational skills required in coordinating a clinical group are complex. Clinical group leader meetings are held biannually where all leaders are encouraged to provide feedback, share positive and difficult elements of their groups, discuss ideas, raise questions, and brainstorm issues with other leaders and the steering committee. Decisions about the ongoing functioning of the Network are made collaboratively with the clinical leaders.

Impact of the web site

The Network's web site has been an invaluable professional support. It has facilitated greater communication and accessibility to information for the SC, clinical leaders, members and general speech and language therapy profession. It has been an invaluable resource to display the function and outcomes of the Network. It is also a public resource which demonstrates that SLTs are actively engaging in EBP through determining clinical questions, searching and critiquing current research and applying this clinical bottom line to practice. As for any web site, it is imperative that the content is current and accurate. This in itself has proven to be challenging. Whilst the support of CIAP staff has been integral to the existence, maintenance and development of the web site, it has proven to be difficult to keep the web site up to date and of high standard.

Impact of the EBP Extravaganza

The annual EBP Extravaganza held gives each group a focus and goal for the year. It allows the leaders to showcase the work of their clinical group and how they are directly applying the evidence into their daily clinical practice. It is the Extravaganza that is the annual 'injection' that helps to keep the Network alive! This is agreed upon to be the largest gathering of clinical SLTs across NSW for the year. Feedback has shown that everyone benefits from other clinical areas presenting on their findings for the year. It is felt that this creates an opportunity for clinicians to keep in touch with clinical updates and changes across the profession in general.

Reflections

The ongoing success of the Network relies on significant commitment, enthusiasm and effort by the SC, clinical group leaders and members. The support of the workplace to be able to provide resources, in terms of time, is integral. There are ongoing challenges in maintaining the momentum and enthusiasm of the Network, but we realize the importance and relevance of evaluating clinical evidence and applying the outcomes.

The NSW Speech Pathology EBP Network has continued to develop since its instigation in 2002. There are now 10 clinical groups with over 200 active members, critically appraising SLT research to endeavour to implement EBP into clinical services. The EBP Network facilitates opportunities for SLTs in NSW to share the responsibility in creating clinical questions, collecting evidence based data, and cooperatively evaluating, discussing and applying it to clinical practice. The Network has provided this framework to build and support a multi-stream clinical system in EBP, and with ongoing support and enthusiasm it is expected that this will continue to evolve.

References

Australian Bureau of Statistics (2008) National regional profile: New South Wales [electronic version]. Retrieved 11h May, 2009 from http://www.abs.gov.au/AUSSTATS/abs@.nsf/9fdb8b444ff1e8e2ca25709c0081a8f9/c673c19381c275afca2571cb000ac6eb!OpenDocument.

Quinn, C., Stevens, A. and Bradd, P. (2002) NSW Speech speech pathology evidence-based practice: Resource package. NSW Speech Pathology Evidence Based Practice Network Resource (unpublished).

Vallino-Napoli, L.D. and Reilly, S. (2004) Evidence-based health care: A survey of speech pathology practice. *Advances in Speech and Language Pathology*, 6 (2), 107–112.

Worrall, L. and Bennett, S. (2001) Evidence-based practice: Barriers and facilitators for speech-language pathologists. *Journal of Medical Speech-Language Pathology*, 9 (2), XI–XVI.

19

Equipping ourselves as evidence-based practitioners: tools and resources for EBP (commentary on Section Four)

Jemma Skeat and Hazel Roddam

An important aspect of moving toward an evidence-based profession will be the tools and resources that we, as clinicians and managers, have available to us, in order to use the evidence in everyday practice. The examples in the previous chapters highlight four different ways that speech and language therapists (SLTs) can equip themselves to embed an EBP approach to their practice, from gathering the views of clients, to developing evidence-based tools, policies and evidence summaries in the form of critically appraised papers and critically appraised topics.

Service users and EBP

We felt it was important to begin this section with a focus on service users. We have emphasized throughout this book that evidence-based practice is built on three things: the research evidence, clinical knowledge and experience, plus the views of clients/patients (Sackett *et al.*, 1996). Thus, approaching our clients and getting their perspectives is essential for us to truly be an evidence-based profession, and Pirkko (Chapter 15) outlines some of the considerations, as well as some of the tools that can be used for this. SLTs have a growing body of work around accessing and using patient views with respect to assessment (e.g. Parr and Byng, 2000), goal setting and outcome evaluation (e.g. Conrad, 1998; Hayhow *et al.*, 2002), and the therapeutic process (e.g. Glogowska and Campbell, 2000; Kagan and Duchan, 2004; Owen *et al.*, 2004), among other things. There are also practical supports in the form of tools that can be used to access client views, even when their communication is restricted, and Pirkko has summarized some of these in her chapter. For some of us, being open to the views of clients presents an ongoing challenge. We are used to presenting ourselves as 'experts', and may feel less than comfortable with asking our clients what they think about what we are planning or what we are doing. Nevertheless, as Pirkko points out, there is a lot at stake if we do not; the effectiveness of our therapy, not to mention the client's satisfaction with what we are doing, may be compromised if we are heading in a different direction to where our clients want to go. A simple starting place for embedding client views within the therapeutic process is suggested by Greenhalgh (1996) who argued that each clinical encounter in the therapeutic setting should include the following elements:

• identifying the area of concern/clinical problem, taking into account the patient's own perception of the problem
• using appropriate tests in order to establish a diagnosis
• taking into account other problems that the patient might have, including risk factors (such as lifestyle and environmental factors, e.g. impact of smoking on voice)
• accessing the available research evidence and evaluating the strength and relevance of this evidence for this patient
• discussing the options with the patient, including the pros and cons of different approaches, and taking this into account when making the final decision.

There are multiple ways that we can access and incorporate patient views, and we hope that Pirkko's chapter, as well as others throughout the book that highlight the ways that SLTs have accessed and used the views of service users (for example, Hannah in Chapter 7 and Sheena and Sarah in Chapter 11), will provide you with some inspiration.

Evidence-based resources that facilitate evidence-based practice

The other chapters in this section have highlighted the development and use of evidence-based resources for practice. Russell (Chapter 16) demonstrates the importance of practical clinical resources that are evidence-based. It is just as important that SLT assessment and treatment materials are based on evidence, as it is that our approaches and service models are. In fact, Bowen *et al.* (2004) argued that without valid, reliable, evidence-based assessment tools, 'the practitioner is unlikely to design an appropriate and effective evidence-based intervention strategy' (p. 509). Angie (Chapter 17) and Tracy, Rachel and Rachelle (Chapter 18) provide examples of tools that summarize and apply the evidence, providing something that is clinically relevant. This may create something that is locally relevant (as in the case of Angie's evidence-based policy), or develop resources that are more broadly applicable (as in the case of the critically appraised topics and papers that Tracy, Rachel and Rachelle's network develops). Evidence-based clinical practice guidelines and protocols are also examples of these resources. While these examples have emphasized the development of these resources, we do not suggest reinventing the wheel if similar resources already exist. In fact, Angie suggests that it is important to take a look around at what other centres are doing, and to consider whether there are existing resources that could be adapted for local needs. The choice of the right form of resource is also critical. In Angie's chapter, the SLT department decided to develop a hospital policy around dysphagia screening, in order to support compulsory training and use of the tool. The key difference between a policy and a clinical practice guideline is often that policies are 'enforceable', with agreed standards that must be followed by employees in the service, while guidelines are not (Hurwitz, 1999). However, the development process for both guidelines and policies is similar. The need for either a guideline, protocol or policy will be dictated largely by local circumstances, as well as the clinical situation or need that prompts the development in the first place.

The resources developed in Tracy, Rachel and Rachelle's chapter were critically appraised topics and critically appraised papers (CATs and CAPs). As the authors describe, CATs and CAPs summarize the evidence around a particular clinical question or topic area, either based on a single paper (CAP) or across several papers (CAT). Brief summaries of the evidence in different clinical areas may be an important approach for facilitating the use of evidence in practice for allied health clinicians (Bennett *et al.*, 2003). They are designed to focus on the 'bottom line' for clinicians and Tracy, Rachel and Rachelle include example forms that they use in their network to guide the development of these resources. Yet the focus for their chapter is not on the development of CATs and CAPs, but on the processes that they use to create and sustain a network of interested clinicians from across New South Wales in Australia, who all contribute to developing these CATs and CAPs. There are many benefits to a 'network' approach such as that described by Tracy, Rachel and Rachelle. The main aim of the network is to allow clinicians to 'share the load' of critical evaluation. By providing a central place for clinicians working in disparate physical locations, the network can bring together those with interests in clinical topics, even very specialized ones in which relatively few clinicians have expertise or interest. With access to the internet, even clinicians in different countries could consider taking the EBP network approach to developing and sharing CATs and CAPs.

Summary

Whatever the approach, the development of evidence-based resources and materials is essential in order to equip ourselves for EBP and to facilitate the practical application of evidence in practice. We hope you have been inspired by some of the examples provided in this section.

References

Bennett, S., Tooth, L., McKenna, K., *et al.* (2003) Perceptions of evidence-based practice: A survey of Australian occupational therapists. *Australian Occupational Therapy Journal*, 50, 13–22.

Bowen, N.K., Bowen, G.L. and Woolley, M.E. (2004) Constructing and validating assessment tools for school-based practitioners. In A.R. Roberts & K. Yeager (eds), *Evidence-based Practice Manual: Research and Outcome Measures in Health and Human Services*. New York: Oxford University Press US, pp. 509–517.

Conrad, C.M. (1998) Outcomes measurement in private practice. In C.M. Frattali (ed.), *Measuring Outcomes in Speech-Language Pathology*. New York: Thieme, pp. 503–513.

Glogowska, M. and Campbell, R. (2000) Investigating parental views of involvement in pre-school speech and language therapy. *International Journal of Language & Communication Disorders*, **35** (3), 391–405.

Greenhalgh, T. (1996) 'Is my practice evidence based?' *British Medical Journal*, **313**, 957–968.

Hayhow, R., Cray, A.M. and Enderby, P. (2002) Stammering and therapy views of people who stammer. *Journal of Fluency Disorders*, **27** (1), 1–17.

Hurwitz, B. (1999) Legal and political considerations of clinical practice guidelines. *British Medical Journal*, **318**, 661–664.

Kagan, A. and Duchan, J. (2004) Consumers' views of what makes therapy worthwhile. In J. Duchan and S. Byng (eds), *Challenging Aphasia Therapies. Broadening the Discourse and Extending the Boundaries*. Hove, UK: Psychology Press, pp. 158–172.

Owen, R., Hayett, L. and Roulstone, S. (2004) Children's views of speech and language therapy in school: Consulting children with communication difficulties. *Child Language Teaching and Therapy*, **20**, 55–72.

Parr, S. and Byng, S. (2000) Perspectives and priorities: Accessing user views in functional communication assessment. In L. Worrall & C. Fratalli (eds), *Neurogenic Communication Disorders. A Functional Approach*. New York: Thieme, pp. 55–66.

Sackett, D.L., Rosenberg, W.M.C., Gray, J.A.M., Haynes, R.B. and Richardson, W.S. (1996) Evidence based medicine: What it is and what it isn't. *British Medical Journal*, **312** (7023), 71–72.

Section Five

Applying evidence to meet clinical challenges

20

A community-based project in rural Sri Lanka

Shalini Felicity Gomesz

Speech Therapist and Teacher Educator, Dr. Peter Bachmann Foundation, Chilaw, Sri Lanka

As sunlight peers through the coconut palms, the birds chirp and the cocks crow, a sleepy hamlet located 96 kilometres away from the bustling city of Colombo slowly comes alive. Most of the villagers are labourers and earn their meager living by picking coconuts, ploughing paddy fields or working in farms. Because of low wages and spiralling cost of living, one member in most families is employed overseas. The village consists of Sinhalese Buddhists who believe that a child with a disability is a sign of punishment for past wrongs, possession by demons, or a deficiency in the horoscope. Remedies are sought through religious and cultural ceremonies. Often the family experiences social stigma and the child is shunned.

When considering developing countries, Sri Lanka is regarded as an 'early pioneer of mainstreaming' (Wertheimer, 1997). Although legislation exists and is expected to play a vital role in safeguarding the rights of children with special educational needs (SEN), implementation is slow and unsystematic. Mainstream schools are able to meet the needs of a very small population. Non-governmental organizations (NGOs) have set up small specialized schools, and these are attended by children with specific learning disabilities who fail in mainstream schools, along with children who have physical, health, sensory, intellectual, and/or behavioural problems.

The majority of teachers in special schools have received the minimum education regarding teaching students with disabilities. The presence of speech and language therapists (SLTs) is rare. Speech and language therapy is at a fledgling stage in Sri Lanka. Less than a hundred SLTs work predominantly in hospitals, while a handful work in educational settings.

One special school for children with disabilities was established in 2003 by a foreign NGO as a community-based rehabilitation project. Under this programme the villagers were required to supply a location and prospective teachers. A wattle and daub building was given by a villager to house the school. The NGO agreed to provide meals for children, resource personnel and study material. The aim of the school is social inclusion. To achieve this goal the school provides education

to develop concrete and practical aspects of learning. In addition, the school promotes community awareness and community involvement in order to encourage
inclusion and to eliminate negative views regarding disability. At the inception,
two teachers were employed to attend to the needs of 10 students, aged 8 to 22
years.

The chief administrator of the school was aware of my interest in working in
rural areas, and my expertise as an SLT and senior lecturer at various universities
and teacher training institutions. He requested that I take on the dual roles of SLT
and teacher educator. I gladly accepted this challenge scheduling a visit per week
to the school. I would spend the first half of the day assessing, planning and
implementing therapeutic goals for students. One teacher would assist me as I
worked with an individual student or a pair. The other teacher, with the help of
a parent, would work with the rest of the students. Once the school day came to
an end, I spent my time educating and training the teachers to expand their teaching skills and implement therapy goals.

Developing verbal communication skills in older children

While communicating with the students I recognized severe limitations in their
verbal communication skills. Students were happy to silently follow instructions
or doze off. They communicated using non-verbal strategies such as eye pointing,
gesture and facial expression. In order to document their communication skills
objectively I had to select an assessment process. Formal assessment was not possible due to the costly nature of standardized tests and their inappropriateness due
to cultural and linguistic differences. For younger students (below 10 years), I was
able to use checklists with relevant age norms. For older students, functional
assessments were carried out by analysing and comparing the communicative
demands placed by the environment and the student's ability to meet these demands.
The skill areas included expressive and receptive language, phonological/articula-
tion and pragmatics skills.

Since most of the students were older than 8 years there was an urgency to
develop effective verbal communication skills swiftly. However, the question
remained, 'what is the evidence for intervention to support language development
in children who are 8 years and beyond?' I undertook a review of the literature,
with this question in mind.

Much of the literature that surfaced dealt with interventions for young children,
and there was little that was specific to older children, particularly in the type of
circumstance that I was seeing at the school. Two studies that appeared similar to
the current context were the examples of 'wild' children (Lenneberg, 1967, cited
in Aitchison, 1998): Amala and Kamala, who were found in India in 1920, having
been reared with wolves, and Genie who was discovered in 1970, having been
confined to a small room under conditions of physical restraint for 14 years.
According to these studies, once found, the children rapidly learned individual
words and concepts but subsequently their progress diminished and stopped altogether. This could be because they had passed the 'critical period' for internaliza-
tion or acquisition of the grammatical and syntactical rules of language. However,

Aitchison (1998) emphasizes that a few cases cannot provide firm proof and rather than specifying an onset or final endpoint to the critical period, it is more suitable to consider a 'sensitive period'; a time early in life when language learning is easier. The ability may reduce gradually thereafter, though not in its entirety. These studies have focused on children totally isolated from human contact. In contrast, the children in Sri Lanka lived in their homes and displayed basic receptive language skills. Aitchison (1998) and others also emphasize that the ability to learn does not cease in its entirety. These factors encouraged me to venture further to unlock the student's potential to communicate verbally.

Literature was scrutinized for possible methods of reaching the goal. Lees and Urwin (1995) advocated designing intervention programmes aimed at developing basic language skills in natural contexts. They suggested focusing on providing a language environment with everyday naturally occurring situations that demand verbal and nonverbal communication. Carlson *et al.* (2000) claimed that overhearing language alone is insufficient for spoken language to emerge. Active verbal interaction between parents, caretakers, teachers and children is vital for the acquisition of language (Gardner, 2006).

The literature thus indicated that a structured, organized programme targeting verbal language development be implemented. Resource constraints and teachers' lack of experience and knowledge required an innovative, low cost and practical action plan. The teachers and I therefore agreed to work collaboratively to devise such a plan. An example of a lesson plan, developed collaboratively and targeting language around animals, is shown in Table 20.1.

After considering the students' responses to traditional classroom teaching, a naturalistic approach was chosen, directly linked to providing an authentic range of opportunities for conversational interactions. Lessons built around familiar themes like 'farm animals' were developed to support advancement of language and communication skills within the context of real life situations and experiences. These lessons were multifaceted and covered all areas of the curriculum. Since teachers had no prior experience of working with students with SEN, I provided training to teachers using suggestions by Ormrod (2000) and others. For example, teachers were encouraged to minimize distractions when talking with students, to listen patiently while students complete their own thoughts, to use picture cues to encourage verbal and non verbal communication, and to follow the children's lead in communication.

Outcomes were measured using pre and post data as outlined in Box 20.1.

Reflections

Implementing a language programme in a rural area of Sri Lanka presented a number of challenges. The need to design assessments and therapeutic material containing colloquial language was time consuming. Blending into the village community, gaining the trust of the villagers, educating and involving families and the community and finding teachers who were capable of carrying on with the work in the future were other challenges faced. Once implemented, evaluating outcomes in naturalistic methods was complicated. We decided to measure multiple outcomes, including language skills and social inclusion (see Box 20.1).

Table 20.1 Example of a lesson based around a theme of 'farm animals'

Thematic unit: Farm animals
Lesson outcomes:
By the end of this theme students will be able to:
  i.   Demonstrate knowledge about farm animals
  ii. Build communal relationships
  iii. Actively communicate

Lesson number	1	2	3	4	5	6	7	8
Environmental studies								
Gathering pre topic knowledge	✓							
Looking at lifecycles (pictures)					✓			
Associating names with features			✓					
Identifying their food				✓				
Discussing differences of farms in other countries via pictures							✓	
Language								
Introducing/learning target words (25)	✓	✓	✓	✓	✓	✓	✓	✓
Listening to a story, answering questions				✓				
Writing a story; whole class								✓
Number								
Counting the different animals on the farm		✓						
Measuring footprints, comparing size and colour of animals		✓						
Purchasing goods						✓		
Science								
Describing physical changes; comparing young with adult animals		✓		✓				
Comparing the ducks and hens eggs and piglets, calves and kids		✓			✓			
Life skills								
Helping feed the animals on the farm. Cleaning their habitats		✓						
Visiting a farm shop						✓		
Making egg sandwiches						✓		
Physical education								
Engaging in competitive games with animal movements			✓					
Music and dancing								
Learning a farm song with appropriate action, moving in response to the tempo of music	✓		✓				✓	
Art and craft								
Making a stuffed animal					✓			
Expressing ideas of the story through drawings								✓

> **Box 20.1   Measuring programme outcomes**
>
> *Assessment of student learning* was conducted during and after each topic (eight lessons), using tasks such as matching, naming and verbal recall. Students and staff enjoyed these activities.
>
> *Oral communication* was assessed through tape recordings of lessons before and after each theme (eight lessons). The once silent hut soon became a hive of activity with children playing and shouting with joy. There were improvements in individual students which exceeded the teachers' expectations.
>
> *Changes in activities in the home and in attitudes of villagers* towards these children were observed. The cookery activity saw many students bring sandwiches, prepared by them, to school the next day; a rare occurrence since they prefer rice. Parents were encouraged include their children when they did their daily grocery shopping. After the field trip parents were more at ease to undertake this challenge. The villagers too began to acknowledge the children with kindness and began to offer their services to teach students cottage industry skills such as weaving, sewing and pottery.

Informal evaluations also helped the teachers to understand the degree of learning.

The programme was conducted with a limited sample of students within a Sinhalese Buddhist cultural context; not wholly representative of the student population with SEN in Sri Lanka. It did not conflict with cultural or religious beliefs. We uncovered the potential for this type of programme. By maintaining a similar sensitivity, the identical approach may be possible in different geographical locations and students of other races, languages and religions. It can therefore be viewed as a base towards designing future intervention programmes. In fact, similar programmes are being implemented in other rural settings with much success.

Attempting to apply the literature around developing language skills in older children posed many challenges. There were few studies available to guide practice with this age group, and even fewer were relevant to a rural population in a developing country. Costly testing material and unsuitability of resources due to cultural and linguistic differences also posed a problem. However, an evidence-based approach was applied by examining the evidence for the development of language skills in older children, and by using recommendations for a structured language programme that provided naturalistic opportunities for verbal language development. All of these evidence-based recommendations were adapted to the needs of the local situation.

References

Aitchison, J. (1998) *The articulate mammal: An introduction to psycholinguistics* (4th edn). London: Routledge.

Carlson, N.R., Buskist, W. and Martin, G.N. (2000) *Psychology: The Science of Behaviour* (European adaptation). Harlow, UK: Allyn & Bacon.

Gardner, H. (2006) Training others in the art of therapy for speech sound disorders: An interactional approach. *Child Language Teaching and Therapy*, 22, 27–46.

Lees, J. and Urwin, S. (1995) *Children with Language Disorders*. London: Whurr.

Ormrod, J.E. (2000) *Educational Psychology: Developing Learners* (3rd edn). Upper Saddle River, NJ: Merrill Prentice Hall.

Wertheimer, A. (1997) *Inclusive Education a Framework for Change: National and International Perspectives*. London: Centre for Studies on Inclusive Education.

21

Supporting communicative participation for children with complex communication needs: how the evidence contributes to the journey

Angela Guidera[1], Catherine Olsson[2] and
Parimala Raghavendra[3]

[1]Assistive Technology Consultant, NovitaTech, South Australia
[2]Profession Leader – Speech Pathology, Novita Children's Services,
South Australia
[3]Manager, Research and Innovation, Division of Research and Innovation,
Novita Children's Services, South Australia

The evidence-based practice (EBP) initiative described in this chapter was undertaken by the speech and language therapy (SLT) department of Novita Children's Services (Novita), an organization based in South Australia. The clinical focus of the SLT department is on augmentative and alternative communication (AAC) and complex dysphagia service delivery. Clients receive services for all communication and swallowing issues prior to school entry but once they have entered school Novita provides services only for AAC, dysphagia and dysarthria needs. Novita is committed to providing EBP. A Clinical Research Department (CRD) was established in 1999 including research senior positions to support the undertaking and implementation of research across the organization.

At the time the initiative described in this chapter was undertaken the SLT department consisted of 17.4 full-time equivalent professional staff. Catherine Olsson was the SLT Clinical Manager and Angela Guidera held the position of Research Senior SLT (a dual research and clinical role). There were a further seven senior SLTs and a number of entry-grade SLTs. Parimala Raghavendra held the position of Clinical Research Manager.

Participation of students who use AAC

Many Novita clients use AAC systems. Students who use AAC systems face a number of challenges to their communicative participation at school, relating to factors such as time constraints and availability of participation opportunities. Communicative participation is defined as 'taking part in life situations where knowledge, information, ideas or feelings are exchanged. ... It involves more than one person and must involve a communicative exchange' (Eadie *et al.*, 2006). Research indicates that there is a large disparity between the needs of children with disabilities and the opportunities usually available in regular classrooms (Carta *et al.*, 1991).

Service provision in schools for children with complex communication needs (CCN) comprised a large proportion of the workload for SLTs at Novita. Services were largely provided directly to children who had limited opportunities and support to interact with educational staff. Evidence was needed to inform development of service delivery models likely to yield the greatest outcomes in relation to communicative participation and to help determine service delivery priorities. Thus, we faced the question: 'what factors influence the participation of children who use AAC in school settings?'

Searching the evidence

Having identified the question as a priority for the SLT service, the Research Senior SLT obtained relevant journal articles by searching databases using key words. Articles relating to children using electronic and non-electronic AAC systems in integrated and special school settings were included. Forty-one articles were identified (see Table 21.1).

A task group was established to support the review and synthesis of the evidence presented across these diverse articles. This group consisted of the Research Senior SLT, the Clinical Research Manager, the SLT Clinical Manager and a number of other SLTs. Articles were distributed for appraisal and the group met regularly to discuss the process. Appraisals were reviewed and collated and the strength of evidence was considered for each of the main factors raised within the literature as being important to communicative participation (e.g. communication partner attitudes/behaviour).

The findings: factors that influence participation

Our review showed that factors which influence participation of students who use AAC systems in school settings include communication partners' attitudes and behaviours, training of school staff, training of peers and direct instruction of the AAC user (Guidera *et al.*, 2002). These factors were considered to have at least a

Table 21.1 Overview of articles appraised

Study type	Number of articles identified
Experimental – Single Subject (SSED)	10
Experimental – Group	8
Meta-analysis of SSED	1
Survey	5
Review	7
Case Study	5
Observational Study	2
Qualitative Study	3

moderate level of evidence. The main types of intervention addressed in the articles included providing communication opportunities, engineering the environment, modelling, using a hierarchy of prompts (for example, expectant look, time delay, command), providing instruction in functional contexts, and using multi-modal communication systems. The findings highlighted a need for an increased focus on training and coaching for communication partners to increase their understanding of the barriers that children who use AAC experience, their expectations for these children and their knowledge, skills and confidence to support communicative participation.

Changing practice to support participation

A key step in implementing our findings was ensuring that they were shared with Novita therapists, managers, and other staff as part of professional development sessions. The information is now presented as part of new SLTs' clinical orientation and has been shared with many clients and families. The results were also used in discussions with strategic partners to support interagency co-ordination and changes in AAC service delivery to improve client outcomes. Meetings were held with government bodies including Disability SA, the Department of Education and Children's Services, and the Flinders University School of Education, to discuss potential changes to service delivery mechanisms and co-ordination around support for children with CCN. Presentations at various national and international AAC and SLT forums (Guidera *et al.*, 2001, 2002; Olsson, 2003) ensured the findings of this review were also shared within the profession.

Our review enabled staff to give families and other stakeholders objective information to assist their decision-making about service delivery needs. Parents' understanding of what is required to support AAC users' participation at school and ability to advocate for appropriate support has been enhanced. In addition, a number of specific service delivery initiatives have been supported through our findings, including the following.

- Establishment of a weekend camp, *Camp Yackety Yack*, and regular *Club Yackety Yack* activities. These focus on building an AAC 'community', supporting networking of children who use AAC and their families, developing children's communicative competence, increasing community awareness and families' and other support people's knowledge about AAC and barriers and facilitators of communicative participation.
- *Songs (and Stories) to Promote Early Language and Learning* (SPELL) projects. These involved workshops for families, service providers and educators about the benefits of songs and stories for learning and communication. They aimed to increase expectations about the potential and abilities of children who use AAC and increase communication partners' knowledge, skills and expertise in providing communication opportunities.
- Establishment of a cross-sector programme focused on provision of training, information and community development in AAC. A *Statewide Complex Communication Needs* service was established in October 2007 for a twelve month period. Training for communication partners was one aspect of the service.

The evidence has also contributed to a number of research initiatives involving SLT staff at Novita. These are shown in Box 21.1.

Box 21.1   Collaborative research initiatives linked to the evidence review

'Participation Profiles of Children with Physical Disabilities with and without Complex Communication Needs: Association between Social Networks, Communication, Activity Engagement and Time Use' (ongoing project at Novita, Raghavendra, Lane, Olsson, Connell and Virgo).

'Professional Learning for School Personnel: Impact on Communication of Students with Severe Disabilities using Speech Generating Devices' (ongoing project at Flinders University, McMillan, Raghavendra, Olsson and Lynch).

'Participation Profiles of Adolescents with and without Complex Communication Needs: The Relationship between Social Networks, Communication and Activity Engagement' (Honours project, McGregor, 2007).

Reflections on barriers and key lessons

The evidence supported a change to existing service delivery processes, which traditionally focused on individually-based needs, for example provision of one-to-one therapy by the SLT. Therefore, our review not only required SLT staff to change their practice, but also other staff (e.g. education staff) to understand and support the changes. We found that presentations and discussions about the findings to therapy providers and education staff were necessary in order to create support for the environmental level interventions that the evidence supported.

We have found that more experienced clinicians are more confident and effective in advocating for a particular model of intervention, when faced with pressure to do things another way. Access to the depth of knowledge, skills and experience available within the department is important, in order to support less experienced staff to provide evidence based service delivery to clients. Remaining barriers include ongoing demands for other interventions, for example, dysphagia management, which impacts on the time available for SLTs to devote to AAC-related training and intervention.

Several lessons have been learned through the experience of implementing the evidence that we identified around participation of children with AAC. The ongoing training in EBP principles available at Novita and the use of evidence appraisal tools was essential to enable staff to critically appraise the research. Evidence is more likely to be implemented into practice if it is reviewed and evaluated by those affected by the outcomes. That is, staff better integrate the information if they are involved in reviewing the research. Involvement in reading and analysing articles helped improve SLTs' skills in critically appraising research. SLTs were supported to prioritize reading and analysis of articles, allowing them time to reflect on their practice within a specific objective framework. We also note that EBP can be a resource intensive process. The processes in place at Novita (e.g. clinician–researcher positions) assisted in our case. Nevertheless, considerable time and effort was involved in training staff in critical appraisal, collating and disseminating the results.

We were able to make changes to practice based on the existing evidence base. It can be difficult to find strong evidence in this area of practice, due to the small, heterogeneous target population and the complex, dynamic nature of the communication process. We were, however, able to identify enough evidence to guide our clinical decision-making and make significant changes to clinical practice in our service.

Dissemination of the findings was a critical part of the process. This is not only a local process, as SLTs working in similar areas face similar problems – thus sharing information about EBP findings through professional and special interest forums will enable more efficacious service delivery across settings and services. Ultimately, integration of evidence, follow up and evaluation takes time and planning. A managed approach that includes ongoing education, support and follow-up is needed.

Where are we now?

We have not formally assessed the impact of the AAC participation review on practice. We plan to undertake evaluation including audits of the site of provision, intervention style and service delivery mechanisms, feedback from SLTs and families plus measurement of SLTs' and others' perceptions of achievement of therapy goals relevant to AAC users' participation at school.

Our observations to date suggest that Novita SLTs understand that AAC participation is significantly impacted by provision of information, training and support that involves the classroom teacher. Staff attempt, wherever possible, to deliver services in this way and there has been an increase in the provision of training for school staff since before the EBP initiative.

Acknowledgements

The authors acknowledge the contributions made by Kylie Opperman, Research Senior Speech Pathologist (who contributed to the later part of the initiative) and other members of the Novita Children's Services' Speech Pathology department.

References

Carta, J., Schwartz, I., Atwater, J. and McConnell, S. (1991) Developmentally appropriate practice: Appraising its usefulness for young children with disabilities. *Topics in Early Childhood Special Education*, **11** (1), 1–20.

Eadie, T., Yorkston, K., Klasner, E., Dudgeon, B., Deitz, J., Baylor, C., Miller, R. and Amtmann, D. (2006) Measuring communicative participation: a review of self-report instruments in speech-language pathology. *American Journal of Speech-Language Pathology*, **15**, 307–320.

Guidera, A., Raghavendra, P. and Olsson, C. (2002) Participation of users in school setting: Research evidence. Proceedings of the Proceedings of the 10th Biennial Conference of the International Society for Augmentative and Alternative Communication, Odense, (pp. 337–338). Toronto: ISAAC.

Guidera, A., Raghavendra, P. and Timko, B. (2001) How can we help children to participate meaningfully in school settings?: Development of an evidence base. Proceedings of the Speech Pathology Australia National Conference, Melbourne. Melbourne: Speech Pathology Australia.

McGregor, S. (2007) Participation profiles of adolescents with and without complex communication needs: The relationship between social networks, communication and activity engagement. Unpublished Honours Thesis, Department of Speech Pathology and Audiology, Flinders University, South Australia, Adelaide.

Olsson, C. (2003) The EBP experiences of an AAC service provider: Diving in deep. *Perspectives on Augmentative and Alternative Communication [Newsletter of Division 12 Special Interest Group of the American Speech-Language-Hearing Association]*, **12** (4), 15–19.

22

Evidence-based diagnosis of speech, language and swallowing following paediatric stroke

Angela Morgan

NHMRC research fellow, Murdoch Childrens Research Institute;
Senior Speech Pathologist, Royal Children's Hospital,
Melbourne, Australia

The Royal Children's Hospital (RCH) is a 300-bed tertiary paediatric hospital in Melbourne, Australia. A child-focused research institute is also housed within the hospital; the Murdoch Childrens Research Institute (MCRI). The co-location of a paediatric hospital and research institute provides the opportunity for clinicians and researchers to work closely together in producing clinical research, in translating research into practice, and in developing evidence-based practice (EBP) initiatives.

The RCH Speech and Language Therapy (SLT) department is lead by a Professor–Director who also heads an MCRI research group. The SLT service consists of three primary streams: structural anomalies, complex medical disorders and acute and rehabilitative neuroscience. The neuroscience stream is the focus for this chapter. Two full-time SLTs work in the acute neurosciences service, and there are two further SLTs (one full-time and one part-time) in rehabilitation. The neurosciences stream largely services children with acquired brain injury, including traumatic brain injury (TBI), brain tumour and stroke. My role crosses both research and clinical areas. I am a research fellow at MCRI and an honorary senior clinician for the RCH SLT department. My clinical and research field of interest is paediatric acquired brain injury.

Assessment in paediatric stroke: the problem

At present, there are no guidelines for SLT management of children with acquired brain injury (e.g. TBI, brain tumour, stroke) within our service. A lack of guidelines or protocols may lead to variability in patient management, likely resulting in unequal patient care, and possibly leading to suboptimal outcomes for some patients. It also leads to a non-systematic approach to record keeping. That is, if there is no mention of dysarthria in a patient record, it is impossible to determine whether the child did not have dysarthria, or whether dysarthria was simply not assessed (e.g. because language abilities were the greater area of assessment need at that time). A systematic approach ensures that all key areas are assessed and documented consistently. In this way we can be confident about the exact prevalence and specific type of communication or swallowing impairment children present with, in addition to how these problems persist or resolve over time. In turn, this data will inform how we should best prioritize, assess and manage a specific population.

The use of evidence-based clinical guidelines reportedly reduces variation in practice, systemizes the quality of care, stimulates research and improves accountability in the diagnosis and treatment of communication disorders (Academy of Neurologic Communication Disorders & Sciences, 2007). The SLT clinical services manager at RCH approached me to work with the clinical team to develop suitable guidelines for the assessment of children with stroke. Thus, there was a need to identify the evidence for the type of speech, language and swallowing disorders occurring in children with stroke. We also needed to determine how and when the team should be assessing and diagnosing these children in order to identify specific targets for intervention.

Examining the evidence

We took three main approaches to examining and accessing the evidence. First, we looked to our own experience and internal audit data; second we looked to the evidence available in other centres (i.e. pre-existing protocols and guidelines); and third we looked to the scientific literature.

Our own experience

Data from a recent SLT stroke service audit helped us examine our local clinical context. In particular, the data were used to identify search terms relevant to our practice for inclusion in the literature review. Local data also provided a systematic way of reflecting upon our current diagnostic approach, including the assessments or screening tools most commonly used, and the timing with which they were applied. We were then able to compare our current practice with that of other centres and the evidence available in the scientific literature.

Evidence from national and international centres

We searched for existing stroke assessment/diagnostic protocols or guidelines used by other national and international centres or established working groups. We were unable to locate protocols/guidelines in Australian, New Zealand or UK centres similar to RCH. An on-line search of other major centres in the UK and the US was also unable to reveal protocols for this population of children (a different finding to the abundance of national and international protocols and guidelines available for children with cleft palate, for example). Only one set of clinical guidelines for children with stroke was identified using an on-line search: the *Stroke in Childhood Clinical Guidelines for Diagnosis, Management and Rehabilitation* (Paediatric Stroke Working Group, 2004). The guidelines related to all aspects of clinical/medical management, and provided general language/

communication information. Interestingly, the only mention of swallowing impairment was a summary of a paper based on the incidence of dysphagia in children with traumatic brain injury (Morgan *et al.*, 2003), not stroke. This finding is in alignment with our own literature search below, indicating that there are no studies focused on dysphagia outcomes for children with stroke. As such, it is likely that the authors of the stroke guidelines were forced to extrapolate data on swallowing outcomes from another paediatric acquired brain injury population.

The scientific literature

We accessed the scientific literature via web-based searches of online databases. MCRI is affiliated with a local university (The University of Melbourne). Whilst RCH has a library, the University library provides access to a wider variety of scientific literature. The team would have experienced difficulty in accessing relevant papers for review without this University association. Further, my research position provided me with dedicated time to perform the literature review. This task would have been challenging for the clinical team who are not allocated time for such tasks in their clinical schedule. Despite our experience that dysphagia is common in the early acute phase post-stroke, no abstracts were identified documenting the existence of swallowing problems in this group. Three abstracts were identified for child stroke and speech disorder (dysarthria, apraxia), and hundreds were identified for child language and stroke. After reading through the abstracts, only twenty-two articles were obtained as being relevant to speech, language or swallowing disorder in paediatric stroke. The literature confirmed that children with stroke may experience a range of speech difficulties (e.g. dysarthria; Gout *et al.*, 2005) and language deficits (e.g. difficulties with word finding, discourse or narrative and speed of information processing; Block *et al.*, 1999; Chapman *et al.*, 2003; Gout *et al.*, 2005). The literature was largely based on low levels of evidence (case studies or cross-sectional case series designs), and was impoverished in terms of identifying specific areas of deficit at specific time points of patient recovery.

Development of a paediatric stroke assessment protocol

Given the impoverished evidence base in this field, particularly for speech and swallowing and in relation to the lack of evidence for critical time periods of resolution of communication and swallowing impairment, the team decided to collect data in this field. Our first goal was to design assessment protocols to be administered systematically at specified time points. The team embarked on this project knowing that this would be a long-term endeavour in order to collect enough evidence to really understand the patterns of diagnosis and prognosis in this group.

The clinical audit data informed us that the current approach to practice was not systematic. Children were assessed with various tools administered at variable time points based on their individual medical and cognitive profile. Anecdotally, this finding is common internationally for clinicians working with the acquired brain injury population. A variable approach is often justified by the heterogeneous nature of this group who present at different ages (e.g. perinatal versus postnatal stroke) with different regions of underlying neural damage, caused by a wide variety of different mechanisms (e.g. ischaemic versus haemorrhagic). However, as noted above, a non-systematic approach not only increases the likelihood of uneven patient care, but also reduces the quality of record keeping, thus limiting the ability to use patient information (e.g. medical records) to identify trends in patient groups, as not all data are systematically reported.

The team meetings therefore initially focused on determining protocols that specified who to assess (e.g. later acquired postnatal stroke versus prenatal stroke), what to assess them with (i.e. assessment batteries to be applied at particular time points), when to assess it (i.e. three time periods as specified below), and where to assess the patients (i.e. acute inpatient ward, inpatient rehabilitation setting, out-patient rehabilitation setting).

The following approach was adopted:

- brief acute informal assessment (within one to two weeks) on the inpatient ward when children are medically stable
- detailed informal and standardized speech, language and swallowing assessment at six to eight weeks on the inpatient ward or as an outpatient
- detailed informal and standardized speech, language and swallowing assessment at twelve months, when many children attend a one-year follow-up outpatient clinic with the rehabilitation team to assess longer-term outcomes.

The protocol was initially implemented on a trial basis, with a focus on evaluating the feasibility and responsiveness of the assessment battery across individuals. The team collected data on two cases using the full protocol and met to discuss the success or shortcomings of the protocol and make changes where required. The perceived benefits included the efficiency of using a predetermined protocol and preprepared assessment packs that were ready to take onto the wards. Whilst the team were wary of using a 'one size fits all' approach to assessment (out of concern that this approach may not meet the needs of individual children), they reported that protocols enabled more time to be spent focused on the child rather than on thinking further about and locating assessments. The team also felt that the systematic approach would improve their record keeping. A negative aspect was that the acute language assessment tool was cumbersome to administer. We are therefore in the process of altering that component of the battery and will pilot the revised protocols on a further two to three patients, meet again, and make any additional modifications. The protocols will then be used on the next ten consecutive patients admitted to RCH. We will also develop data sheets to ensure a standardized approach to reporting of results in the patient's file. A database will be developed in order to enter this data for successful monitoring and evaluation of outcomes. The team will continue to meet regularly, practicing an ongoing action research cycle to further develop our protocols, see Figure 22.1.

Reflections and key lessons

The key barrier to implementation was the behavioural change needed to alter existing practices, specifically the use of a systematic assessment protocol at specified time points rather than using a case-by-case approach. Lively discussion

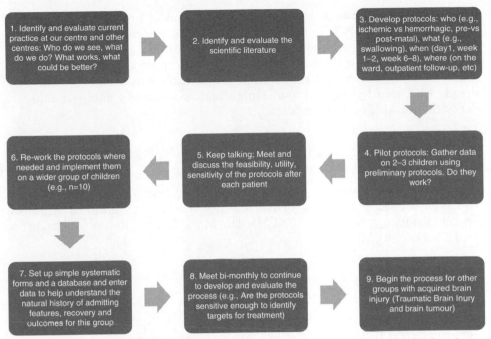

Figure 22.1 Flowchart of approach used in the creation and ongoing evaluation of evidence-based protocols for stoke assessment at RCH.

occurred at protocol development meetings, particularly around the need to be responsive to the children's needs at appropriate time periods. By acknowledging issues and concerns, and discussing the evidence, we were able to come to consensus to trial the new approach.

A number of key opportunities facilitated the implementation of change in our service. A more formalized acute paediatric stroke service had recently been launched at RCH, providing the perfect context for evaluating and improving current practice. The head medical consultant of the stroke service had strong working relationships with SLT team members and supported this initiative. The head of the clinical SLT service was also supportive of the endeavour. Thus, we had the authority to make changes to practice, and the clinical impetus to focus on care for this population; both of these factors supported this initiative.

In terms of evaluation, we did not predetermine measurable outcomes for evaluating the change associated with implementing protocols for assessment of stroke. However two broad areas for potential improvement in clinical practice were identified in an *ad-hoc* fashion during the piloting process: (i) improvement in the systematic reporting of communication/swallowing disorder; and (ii) increased efficiency due to predetermined protocols. Areas that will be targeted once we have finalized the stroke protocols and implemented these across the service include patient outcomes (e.g. decreased average length of time to achieving a full oral diet) and/or service delivery outcomes (e.g. increased referrals from the medical team, earlier assessment and screening of communication and swallowing problems, earlier discharge from SLT services).

Due to the implementation of the stroke assessment protocol, assessment of paediatric stroke at RCH is now driven by existing evidence (for example, that these children have speech and language difficulties). We are also adding to the evidence through clear documentation of our assessment and diagnosis of these children. While we are still trialling our protocol for assessment, benefits have already been seen by staff, who are embracing the systematic approach and efficiency that this brings to client care.

Acknowledgements

Sincere thanks to: Maria Fassoulakis, Flora Haritou, Sue Morse, Justine Slattery, Samantha Heriz, Jane Mah, Bernadette O'Connor, and Elizabeth Murdoch (Speech Pathology Department, RCH); Dr. Mark Mackay (Head of Paediatric Stroke Service, RCH).

References

Academy of Neurologic Communication Disorders & Sciences (2007) What is evidence-based practice? Retrieved 12 July 2008 from http://www.ancds.org/

Block, G.W., Nanson, J.L. and Lowry, N.J. (1999) Attention, memory and language after paediatric ischemic stroke. *Child Neuropsychology*, 5 (2), 81–91.

Chapman, S.B., Max, J.E., Gamino, J.F., McGlothlin, J.H. and Starr, N.C. (2003) Discourse plasticity in children after stroke: age at injury and lesion effects. *Paediatric Neurology*, 29 (1), 34–41.

Gout, A., Seibel, N., Rouvière, C., *et al.* (2005) Aphasia owing to subcortical brain infarcts in childhood. *Journal of Child Neurology*, 20 (12), 1003–1008.

Morgan, A., Ward, E., Murdoch, B., Kennedy, B. and Murison, R. (2003) Incidence, characteristics and predictive factors for dysphagia after pediatric traumatic brain injury. *Journal of Head Trauma Rehabilitation*, 18 (3), 239–251.

Paediatric Stroke Working Group (2004) *Stroke in Childhood Clinical Guidelines for Diagnosis, Management and Rehabilitation*. London: Clinical Effectiveness and Evaluation Unit, Royal College of Physicians.

23

Working with a dysfluent three-year-old from a bilingual family

Patricia Oksenberg

Speech and Language Therapist, Levallois-Perret, France

I am a speech and language therapist (SLT) with an independent practice in a suburb of Paris. I specialize in disorders of fluency and have recently completed specialist training at the Georges Pompidou European Hospital in Paris in this area. I currently work with children, teenagers or adults who present a variety of stammering difficulties.

Stammering is currently understood to be a communication disorder (Montfrais-Pfauwadel, 2000), which is probably genetically/biologically driven (Shapiro, 1999; Watkins, 2008). There are both overt and covert symptoms of stammering (Sheehan, 1970). Overt symptoms are what you hear when communicating with a dysfluent speaker, whereas covert symptoms refer to the feelings, attitudes and thoughts that are brought on by the dysfluency. SLTs need to address both aspects of the disorder in order to best help the person with a stammering difficulty. In the preschool years, prevalence of stuttering is around 2.4% (Yairi and Ambrose, 2005), and this prevalence decreases as children grow older, with around 0.5% of teenagers affected (0.8% boys and 0.2% girls) (Craig *et al.*, 2002).

In France, preschool dysfluency is traditionally managed using a family-focussed approach (Chabert *et al.*, 2005). This approach consists of giving advice to parents to allay anxieties, and suggesting ways to change and improve the family's communication styles. Recent research has shown that such approaches are effective in managing stammering (Millard *et al.*, 2008). Parents' feelings have to be considered, as well as what they do physically when their child is stammering, for example, whether they look away (Chabert *et al.*, 2005). Other common clinical approaches to the management of preschool dysfluency include behavioural approaches such as the Lidcombe programme (Onslow *et al.*, 2003), and the Palin PCI approach (Kelman and Nicholas, 2008).

This chapter will focus on a recent case of stammering, which presented a clinical problem for which I needed to seek guidance from the research evidence. This was a case of stammering in the context of bilingualism. It will centre on my clinical input with a child named Alex, who was from a bilingual (French–Italian speaking) family. The key psycholinguistic, psychosocial and therapeutic factors that need to be considered when working with preschool children who stutter, and who have bilingual family backgrounds, were investigated.

Stammering and bilingualism: the case of Alex

Alex was referred to me by the Trousseau Children's Hospital in Paris in October 2005 because of his early stuttering difficulties. I saw Alex for an initial assessment of his fluency skills and needs at the age of three years and seven months. Prior to this, Alex had already been seen by two SLTs. His parents had received advice about communicating with Alex, yet his parents told me that the stutter persisted and became worse. It was also clear that previous SLT input had not viewed the presenting stuttering difficulties in relation to the bilingual French–Italian speaking home background.

The dysfluency was starting to have significant psycholinguistic and psychosocial implications for Alex and his family. Alex was blocking at the start of words and was showing associated secondary dysfluency features such as disrupted breathing patterns, lip movements prior to speech and reduced eye contact in interactions. Alex's mother, Julia, was becoming increasingly concerned about her son's speech difficulties. She also reported stressful events in the family, such as a recent miscarriage. Every significant family event may have an impact on children's fluency (Chabert *et al.*, 2005).

Alex's language background

Julia is an Italian who speaks French fluently as her second language but with a marked Italian accent. Julia spoke a combination of the two languages with Alex at home. Alex's father, Leo, only speaks French with Alex. Leo was also very anxious about Alex's stammering difficulties. He also reported that he felt guilty because Alex's dysfluency began whilst Alex was staying with his French grandparents for ten days.

Reviewing the evidence

I decided that I should consider the research evidence for the potential influence of bilingualism to exacerbate fluency difficulties in childhood and to make the dysfluency more challenging to treat and manage. In view of the complexities of this case, I also felt that it was important to record a detailed case history, including Alex's and his parents' view of the problem. These enquiries would comprise the first two strands of evidence-based practice (EBP) – the research evidence, plus the patient's perspectives of the problem. The third strand of the EBP model is the clinician's expert judgement in planning the most appropriate intervention and case management (Sackett *et al.*, 1997).

The research literature indicated that there may be a link between bilingualism and stammering. Specifically, children using two or more languages in the home may be more likely to stammer (Howell *et al.*, 2009; Van Borsel *et al.*, 2001). It is useful to consider stammering and bilingualism in relation to the 'demands and capacities' model (Starkweather, 1987; Starkweather and Ridener-Gottwald,

1990). This model proposes that dysfluent behaviours occur when the demands placed on the child begin to outweigh their capacities. Thus, in the clinic, SLTs often see the onset of dysfluency when a child begins to increasingly use a second language.

Case history

The initial case history contained a lot complex and sensitive information related to the onset of Alex's stammering difficulty. Consequently, there were lengthy discussions with both parents during the initial assessment and consultation. We talked about the impact of bilingualism on Alex's stammering, and the potential difficulty of Alex juggling three phonologic systems: French and Italian, plus French spoken with an Italian accent, as spoken by his mother.

Clinical observations

A complete assessment to examine all aspects of Alex's language functioning was completed shortly after the first fluency assessment. Initial clinical observations and relevant standardized tests indicated that Alex was a lively child and he had a good language level for a child of his age. His phonological and articulation skills were also largely age appropriate. More careful listening, however, showed that Alex often produced the /s/ sound with a lateral quality. The word 'yes' ('*oui*' in French) was always pronounced 'si' as in Italian (the word '*si*' exists in French but the meaning is not the same as 'yes'). At times, hesitation between two languages caused Alex's speech to become completely blocked. This occurred primarily when Alex began to speak in Italian, and then made an effort to switch to French.

Alex's performance on certain sections of the language assessment battery highlighted that he was experiencing occasional word-finding difficulties. The assessment also showed that Alex often found it difficult to judge and interpret different facial expressions. For example, on one of the test items, Alex found it difficult to judge whether a character's face was happy or sad. During the test, it is significant to note that Alex's mother had a very fixed facial expression when he was stammering. It also appeared that Alex did not look at his mother whilst he was speaking.

It was during the second assessment session that I began to understand the significant impact of the bilingual home context on the stammering and the potential negative impact on the proposed treatment plan. During the session Julia spoke Italian for directive language, such as: 'Help the lady to put away her parcels', or 'Don't pick up the pencils!' In these situations, Alex did not say anything and did not look at his mother. I noticed that he did not like it when Julia spoke Italian in front of me.

Decisions about management for Alex

I proposed having a regular session with one of the parents and Alex once a month. Alongside these sessions, we discussed options for reducing the demands placed on Alex's language. Alex's mother wanted to give Alex the opportunity to be bilingual, but she was aware that it was very important for Alex to speak French well. She did not insist on the use of Italian very thoroughly. After discussing my observations with Julia, particularly about Alex's reaction to her use of Italian, she decided to speak only French with Alex at home until the next appointment. When only one language was used with Alex at home, his stammering began to noticeably reduce. I then asked Alex which he preferred, and without any blocking or hesitation he said 'I like it when Mummy speaks French'.

Outcomes

Both parents reported that Alex experienced fewer hesitations when he knew that only one language was spoken at home. Alex didn't try to check his speech anymore. He spoke without stress, without any hesitation. Given such improvements, Julia was now able to look at her son when he spoke. After two sessions, Alex was speaking fluently. We therefore decided to stop the sessions and to review again in six months.

I saw Alex in clinic for a review six months later. After a period of only speaking French at home, Alex had started to speak Italian. He accepted the idea that his mother would speak to him in Italian. Very quickly, he answered fluently in Italian. Now Alex is bilingual. Currently, there are no more instances of blocking, only a few residual dysfluencies but without tension. His eye contact is good and he is now better able to judge and interpret the facial expressions of others.

Reflections on applying the evidence to Alex's case

An application of the research evidence to the case of Alex would suggest that the bilingual home context together with his 'shaky' phonological system, word finding difficulties and a reduced ability to analyse and interpret facial expressions were all contributing factors in his early dysfluent phase. In this case a traditional approach alone was not enough as all of the contributing factors needed to be considered and therapeutically managed where appropriate. Indeed it is becoming increasingly recognized in the clinical literature that all other aspects of the child's communicative functioning (speech, phonology, language and social communication) need to be addressed in order to improve the child's fluency levels (Kelman and Nicholas, 2008). Additionally, through my reading of the literature and observations during assessment sessions, it became apparent that one part of the treatment would need to address the second-language load on Alex.

It was not easy as a therapist to tell Alex's mother to speak only French to her son when I knew she was Italian. This is not what I usually recommend as it is generally easier and more natural for a mother to convey her emotions in her first language rather than in an additional language. It was clear, however, that when French became the only language spoken at home, a considerable amount of tension was removed for Alex. In this case, clinical decision-making regarding the course of intervention for Alex was based on research evidence, my own clinical experience, and the views of the family, particularly Alex who expressed a preference for his mother to speak French.

Acknowledgements

I am grateful to Simon Henderson (UK), for his helpful comments on drafts of my chapter as well as assistance with translation. Thanks are also due to my teacher and mentor, Nadia Brejon Teitler (France).

References

Chabert, M., Marvaud, J., Simon, A.-M. and Vidal-Giraud, H. (2005) *Bégaiement : intervention préventive précoce chez le jeune enfant [Stuttering: Early preventive intervention for young children]*. Paris: APB Association Parole Bégaiement.

Craig, A., Hancock, K., Tran, Y., Craig, M. and Peters, K. (2002) Epidemiology of stuttering in the community across the entire lifespan. *Journal of Speech, Language and Hearing Research*, **45**, 1097–1105.

Howell, P., Davis, S.R. and Williams, R. (2009) The effects of bilingualism on stuttering during late childhood. *Archives of Disability in Childhood*, **94**, 42–46.

Kelman, E. and Nicholas, A. (2008) *Practical Intervention for Early Childhood Stammering: Palin PCI Approach*. London: Speechmark.

Millard, S.K., Nicholas, A. and Cook, F.M. (2008) Is parent–child interaction therapy effective in reducing stuttering? *Journal of Speech, Language and Hearing Research*, **51**, 636–650.

Montfrais-Pfauwadel, M-C. (2000) *Un manuel du bégaiement [A handbook of stuttering]*. Marseille: SOLAL.

Onslow, M., Packman, A. and Harrison, E. (2003) *The Lidcombe Program of Early Stuttering Intervention: A Clinician's Guide*. Austin, TX: Pro-Ed.

Sackett, D.L., Richardson, W.S., Rosenberg, W.M.C. and Haynes, R.B. (1997) *Evidence-based Medicine: How to Practice and Teach EBM*. London: Churchill Livingstone.

Shapiro, D.A. (1999) *Stuttering Intervention*. Austin, TX: Pro-Ed.

Sheehan, J.G. (1970) *Stuttering: Research and Therapy*. New York: Harper and Row.

Starkweather, C.W. (1987) *Fluency and Stuttering*. Englewood Cliffs, NJ: Prentice-Hall.

Starkweather, C.W. and Ridener-Gottwald, S. (1990) The demands and capacities model II: Clinical applications. *Journal of Fluency Disorders*, **15**, 143–157.

Van Borsel, J., Macs, E. and Foulon, S. (2001) Stuttering and bilingualism: A review. *Journal of Fluency Disorders*, **26**, 179–205.

Watkins, K.E. (2008) Les bases neurales du bégaiement [The neural basis of stuttering]. Presentation made to the Association Parole Bégaiement. Ecole Normale Supérieure (National University).

Yairi, E. and Ambrose, N. (2005) *Early Childhood Stuttering*. Austin, TX: Pro-Ed.

24

Supporting parents and teachers in managing autism: an example of an evidence-informed model for assessment and intervention

Anneli Yliherva

Speech and Language Therapist, Faculty of Humanities,
Logopedics, University of Oulu, Finland

In Finland, the screening of developmental disorders is usually made in health care centres, mainly at the child welfare clinic by a public health nurse. Nurses refer children with suspected autism for further evaluations, for example, to a psychologist or speech and language therapist (SLT). If needed, a child may be referred again to specialist health care (usually a university hospital), where the diagnostic evaluation of childhood autism is made in a multi-professional team, usually in the child neurological ward. At the University Hospital of Oulu, I worked in a multi-professional team where the diagnosis of autism was mainly based on examinations of a child neurologist, psychologist and SLT. Medical and other evaluations often supported the diagnosis as well.

This chapter describes the case of Mary, a young girl with autism. I will use this case to show how we have approached the evidence at University Hospital in two areas:

- creating an evidence-based model of assessment and intervention that focuses on supporting parents and education professionals (e.g. day care staff) to enable carry-over of treatment into the child's everyday environment;
- the use of evidence-based interventions, such as the picture exchange communication system (PECS) which is reported to facilitate language development in people with autism.

Supporting parents and teachers

As autistic children's main problems are those concerning speaking and communication, speech and language therapy treatment is usually the primary intervention at preschool age. It is a huge challenge to support family, and others in the child's environment, to cope with a child with autism in everyday life, and an additional challenge for therapists to get evidence-based knowledge about the possible effect of treatment in these situations. In a review of the evidence for treat-

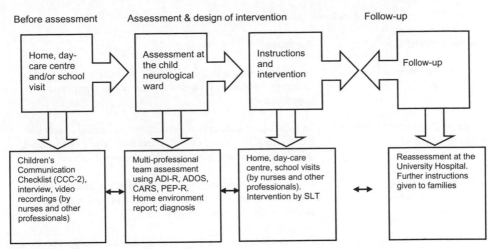

Figure 24.1 Model of assessment and intervention for children with autism at the University Hospital of Oulu.

ment of childhood autism, Yliherva and Olsén (2007) found that individual therapy alone is not the most effective method; treatment implemented in everyday life is needed. However, many times in clinical work there exists a barrier between professionals in special health care and people in child's environment, such as parents and kindergarten teachers in day-care. This is why we wanted to create a protocol (see Figure 24.1), which would outline the process for assessment and intervention with a focus on supporting the child's parents as well as professionals in day care centre. The aim was to change the assessment and follow-up of treatment to become more systematic and effective. In particular, visits by hospital staff such as SLTs to the child's home and child care environment, before and after examination time were emphasized. This evidence-based model was tested in practice at the University Hospital of Oulu, to examine its potential effectiveness.

The case of Mary

Mary was referred to the University Hospital at the age of three years, eight months, following a history of problems in language development and social interaction which were observed first by her parents. Mary had problem behaviours, especially at home but also at day-care. According to aetiological investigations there was no reason for the problems in social interaction and communication. The diagnosis of childhood autism was confirmed and intervention started at the age of three years, ten months. The follow-up of intervention lasted until Mary was four years, six months: a total of eight months.

Assessment

In Finland the diagnostic criteria for childhood autism is based on ICD-10 (World Health Organization, 1999) or DSM-IV (American Psychiatric Association, 2000).

Table 24.1   Assessment methods used for diagnosing childhood autism

Assessment	Purpose
Children's Communication Checklist-2 (CCC-2)	To differentiate the diagnosis of autism from one of specific language impairment. Parents or caregivers complete the questionnaire
Autism Diagnostic Interview Revised (ADI-R)	To assess problems in communication and social interaction (based on ICD-10 and DSM-IV) and their effect on a child's/adult's environment using parent/caregiver interview
Autism Diagnostic Observation Schedule (ADOS)	To assess problems in child's communication and social interaction (based on ICD-10 and DSM-IV) using play situations and/or conversation
Childhood Autism Rating Scale (CARS)	To assess degree of autism, problems in communication and social interaction and in general development using parent interview
Psycho-Educational Profile Revised (PEP-R)	To assess development in seven areas (imitation, perception, fine and gross motor skills, verbal and nonverbal skills, visuomotor coordination) and deviant behaviour in interaction, emotional expression, play and interests in a structured situation

The most important areas in setting the diagnosis of autism are communication and social interaction. A battery of assessments (see Table 24.1) are used at our hospital, and these were placed into the new process for assessment and intervention that is outlined in Figure 24.1.

In Mary's case, we did not need to complete the CCC-2 (Bishop, 2003) because there was no need for making a differential diagnosis between autism and specific language impairment (SLI).

In keeping with our process for assessment and treatment, the first step in Mary's assessment was a visit to the home and the day-care centre, in this case, carried out by a nurse. She interviewed the parents and staff at the day-care centre to get information about Mary's behaviour in different situations. Following this, Mary and her parents attended the hospital for formal assessment. The hospital psychologist and SLT together performed the ADI-R (Lord *et al.*, 1994) and the ADOS (Lord *et al.*, 2000) which were both video-recorded. Other members of the multi-professional team, such as nurses and other therapists, performed the CARS (Schopler *et al.*, 1998) and the PEP-R (Schopler *et al.*, 1990). A summary of all the assessments and all the information gathered earlier by the nurse from Mary's environment was used in clinical decision–making, and a diagnosis of autism was made. After this, further home and day-care centre visits were done again by a nurse and a SLT. The aim was to systematically teach the parents and day-care staff how to support Mary's communication and social skills in daily activities.

Intervention

In Mary's case the main object of intervention was to improve her communication and social interaction. The therapy method used by the SLT was PECS (Bondy and Frost, 2002), which was chosen because it has been reported to be effective in supporting children to initiate communication, for example, requesting (Yoder and Stone, 2006). In many cases lack of speech or problems in communication are the main causes for behavioural problems that make barriers for normal social life. We also implemented a method specifically designed for children with autism called The TEACCH (Treatment and Education of Autistic and related Communication-Handicapped Children) programme (Schopler and Mesibov, 1995) to structure the environment visually at Mary's home and day-care centre. Weekly direct intervention was implemented, and parents and staff at the day-care centre were given support and instructions to further implement the intervention programme. Mary also had access to a teacher's aide/assistant who further supported the implementation of the programme, which lasted for eight months. Mary was also practising different skills based on her profile in the PEP-R (e.g. gross and fine motor skills) on each day with her aide/assistant or parents.

Outcome after intervention

Mary's performance was followed up by reassessment after the eight month period of intervention. We found that she had made improvements in her behaviour, particularly in social interaction as measured by the ADOS. Additionally, her fine and gross motor skills as measured by the PEP-R, had improved. There was no change in communication as measured by the ADOS; however the overall change indicated by the ADOS showed that Mary's autistic features were alleviated after the intervention. We have had the same kind of experience using PECS in the case of an adult autistic person. Specifically, after using the PECS this client's active initiations in communication and active social interaction were more frequent, but these positive benefits were difficult to measure using formal assessments.

While these objective improvements were important, we were also interested in the reports of parents and day-care staff about Mary's behaviour and skills in the 'real world', as this had been a target of the intervention. In Mary's case, problem behaviour had decreased at day-care centre, according to teacher's comments. Parents were asked later (by telephone interview) how they felt about the intervention program and the answer was that their family satisfaction was better than before the intervention started, even though Mary's problem behaviour remained about the same at home.

According both to parental comments and our experiences working with Mary, our approach to clinical assessment and intervention, which emphasized the environmental factors, was functioning well in Mary's case. The intensive follow-up during the intervention helped people in Mary's environment to cooperate better with her. Visits at home and day-care centre supported those working with her in everyday life. We found that it was worthwhile to support parents and professionals during the intervention to reach the aims better than just to leave them work by themselves.

Reflections on using evidence to guide assessment and intervention for Mary

Our aim was to change assessment and intervention of autistic children in the organization, based on evidence. Using evidence-based practice in clinical work gives a systematic view to the work and gives an opportunity to consider how to do the assessment and intervention more effectively. It is important that subjective reports are included systematically, so that we can examine the subtle changes that assessment tools sometimes miss. For example, our use of the PECS with Mary did not facilitate her communication; however, there were positive benefits for everyday life in her family and day-care centre.

Acknowledgements

I want to thank Mary and her parents for giving a permission to introduce her case, the head of the Department of Pediatrics and Adolescence, MD, PhD Päivi Tapanainen for giving support to this initiative and professor Irma Moilanen and MD Marja-Leena Mattila for allowing us to use Finnish translations of the ADI-R and the ADOS in our clinic. Finally I want to express my warm thanks to my colleague, neuropsychologist Merja Ervasti, and the neurological team at the University Hospital of Oulu. It has been a pleasure to work with the team.

References

American Psychiatric Association (2000) *Diagnostic and Statistical Manual of Mental Disorders (DSM-IV)*. Washington: American Psychiatric Publishing.

Bishop, D.V.M. (2003) *The Children's Communication Checklist* (2nd edn). London: The Psychological Corporation.

Bondy, A. and Frost, L. (2002) The picture exchange communication system. *Focus on Autistic Behaviour*, **9**, 1–19.

Lord, C., Risi, S., Lambrecht., L., *et al.* (2000) The Autism Diagnostic Observation Schedule – Generic: A standard measure of social and communication deficits associated with the spectrum of autism. *Journal of Autism and Developmental Disorders*, 30, 205–223.

Lord, C., Rutter, M. and LeCouteur, A. (1994) Autism Diagnostic Interview – revised: a revised version of diagnostic interview for caregivers of individuals with possible pervasive developmental disorders. *Journal of Autism and Developmental Disorders*, **24**, 659–668.

Schopler, E. and Mesibov, G. (1995) *Learning and Cognition in Autism* (2nd edn). New York: Plenum Press.

Schopler, E., Reichler, R., Bashford, A., Lansing, M.D. and Marcus, L.M. (1990) *Individualized Assessment and Treatment for Autistic and Developmentally Disabled Children. Vol 1. Psychoeducational Profile Revised (PEP-R)*. Austin, TX: Pro-Ed.

Schopler, E., Reichler, R. and Renner, B. (1998) *The Childhood Autism Rating Scale: CARS*. Los Angeles: Western Psychological Sciences.

World Health Organization (1999) *International Classification of Diseases (ICD)* (2nd Finnish edn). Stakes, Helsinki: WHO.

Yliherva, A. and Olsén, P. (2007) Mitä tiedämme lapsuusiän autismista [The treatment of early childhood autism]. *Finnish Medical Journal*, 33, 2859–2865.

Yoder, P. and Stone, W. (2006) Randomized comparisons of two communication interventions for preschool children with autism spectrum disorders. *Journal of Consulting and Clinical Psychology*, 74, 426–435.

25

Communication therapy on the Stroke Care Unit

Daniel De Stefanis and Gracie Tomolo

Speech Pathologists, Royal Melbourne Hospital, Melbourne, Australia

The Royal Melbourne Hospital – City Campus (RMH) in Victoria is a 350-bed acute metropolitan tertiary referral teaching hospital. Its clinical services supply the north and west of metropolitan Melbourne and provide specialist services to greater Victoria. At the time of the initiative described in this chapter, both authors worked whin the speech and language therapy (SLT) team at RMH, which admits over 800 people with stroke per year with this figure increasing annually. The 16-bed capacity Stroke Care Unit (SCU) is staffed by a multidisciplinary team, including one full-time SLT. Within the hospital, evidence-based practice (EBP) is prioritized and supported through a number of initiatives. An on-site library includes relevant books, journals, electronic access to databases and online journals. There is also librarian support for evidence-based searches.

At RMH, dysphagia assessment and management is generally prioritized above communication therapy as untreated dysphagia is associated with both malnutrition and aspiration pneumonia (Smithard *et al.*, 1996). In 2007, the SLT working on the SCU became concerned that clients with communication disorders requiring therapy would often wait in the acute hospital for further medical investigations or for a transfer to their discharge destination without access to communication rehabilitation. In early 2007, the National Stroke Foundation (NSF) Acute Care Guidelines (NSF, 2007) were distributed, which included evidence-based guidelines for the treatment of communication disorders. These guidelines stated, 'patients with communication difficulties should be treated as early and as frequently as possible' (p. 34). This specific guideline was based on two systematic reviews, representing strong (level I) and moderate (level III-2) evidence. This guideline, coupled with the therapist's concern became the impetus for this small EBP project.

Investigating the evidence for early communication therapy

In order to investigate this area further, a clinical question was formulated: 'In clients with stroke related communication disorders, does therapy in the acute and

174

subacute setting versus therapy in the subacute setting alone lead to improved eventual communication outcomes?'

We searched online databases (MedLine, CINAHL and PubMed) for evidence to answer this question. An immediate issue became clear around defining what was meant by 'acute' or 'early' therapy. Many articles defined this as 'within the first three months post-stroke', which did not match our need to find evidence specific to the acute setting. At RMH clients suffering from stroke have a length of stay of an average of eight days (Weir and Cadilhac, 2007).

We found that there was a scarcity of research addressing our specific clinical question. While some articles describing early dysphasia therapy have been published, no articles comparing therapy in the acute and subacute setting with therapy in the subacute setting alone were located. Furthermore, no articles focusing on dyspraxia, dysarthria or cognitive communication disorders were available. We revised our clinical question to explore early versus late rehabilitation for language disorders following stroke. This question was relevant to the problem that we had identified, but did not limit studies to only those considering 'acute' versus 'subacute'.

Six articles were identified as being relevant to the issue of early versus late rehabilitation for language disorders following stroke. Two articles (Enderby et al., 1987; Hartman, 1981) referred to 'spontaneous recovery': a process by which stroke survivors with communication disorders (or other physical and cognitive-perceptual disorders) tend to recover in the early period post stroke without intensive therapy and explained how this could be a confounding factor in investigations regarding very early rehabilitation. Two other articles (Holland and Fridriksson, 2001; Lalor and Cranfield, 2004) discussed dysphasia management in the acute care setting. Holland and Fridriksson (2001) suggested language intervention in the form of a supportive role with regular assessments of functional performance. Lalor and Cranfield (2004) identified that clients with dysphasia in the acute setting were appropriate for early rehabilitation; however, few received therapy due to caseload demands. The final two articles (Bhogal et al., 2002; Robey, 1998) were meta-analyses addressing dysphasia therapy. These meta-analyses were the articles used to formulate the NSF guidelines and as such were considered highly influential in our review. Robey suggested that clients with dysphasia who were treated displayed significantly more improvement than those who were not. He further concluded that the effect of therapy was greater in the earlier phases post-stroke. Both reviews suggested that high intensity therapy produced better language outcomes, and Robey specified that clients required a minimum of two hours of therapy per week.

Thus, the existing evidence suggested that language therapy should be implemented in the early phases post-stroke, and that, if possible, a high intensity approach should be implemented.

Implementing the evidence: communication therapy on the SCU

A plan was implemented to increase the availability of communication therapy to clients with dysphasia post-stroke. Medical, allied health and nursing staff were encouraged to refer clients with suspected communication difficulties to the SLT.

Communication was assessed by the SLT using a locally developed tool. If a language deficit was noted and the client was deemed appropriate (that is, medically stable and able to remain alert for periods of at least 15 minutes), a tailored therapy programme was commenced immediately. Programmes included:

- provision of augmentative and alternative communication (AAC) options
- provision of communication strategies to clients, family members and the multidisciplinary team
- impairment-based therapy (e.g. semantic categorization).

Barriers to early communication therapy

While there was evidence to support the implementation of early communication therapy on the SCU, there were a number of barriers to be overcome in order to change practice. They included the following.

- *Competing priorities*: in the acute setting, the assessment and management of dysphagia, communication assessment, and discharge planning have traditionally been seen as the primary roles of the SLT, leaving little time for planning and implementation of therapy programmes.
- *Therapy resources*: The majority of the department's dysphasia therapy resources were difficult to obtain quickly as they were located on another site. A range of different activities were needed in order to provide well-targeted therapy sessions for patients whose impairment is rapidly changing in the early phase post-stroke.
- *Clinical expertise and experience*: Although a system for supervision is well established at RMH, the SLT engaged in the stroke and neurology caseload is traditionally a rotating acute grade one position (i.e. up to six years post-graduation). Thus, the SLT had varying degrees of experience in formulating therapy programmes.

A number of actions were discussed and executed, in order to overcome these difficulties. Strategies were implemented to ensure that workloads did not significantly increase. For example, clients who were able to self-correct were provided with activities to be completed independently, with the SLT reviewing the results and making changes to the programme as appropriate. If the client's family were regularly available they were encouraged to assist with therapy activities and were taught strategies to facilitate more effective communication with the client. Fortunately, the department had access to an allied health assistant (AHA), who was employed for four hours per week. The AHA assisted with implementing therapy tasks and provided opportunities for the client to practise using any AAC systems. With a combination of SLT, AHA, family- and client-directed therapy sessions, increases in therapy provision were possible.

In order to make therapy materials more accessible, a stock-take of available therapy material was undertaken. Activities that were considered appropriate were grouped into a therapy folder and stored on the SCU. Activities in the folder were arranged in a hierarchical fashion to allow for easy 'step-up/step-down' contingencies. Low-tech AAC systems were created and copies were made for use with future clients.

Finally, support for the SLT was provided through clinical supervision and access to appropriate professional development activities. Additionally, the SLT found the departmental daily 30-minute caseload allocation meeting beneficial in discussing and developing appropriate dysphasia therapy programmes for clients.

Evaluating change

Therapy was conducted with around ten clients over a four month period on the SCU. There were no quantitative measures taken; however, some positive outcomes were observed. Clients who were selected for early communication therapy were highly motivated. Often clients and their families worked together to achieve the common language therapy goal. This was felt to impact positively on client's mood, morale and satisfaction. Where clients received early language therapy on the SCU, the SLT detected an increase in their insight and awareness of language deficits. This was also felt to contribute to professional satisfaction, as SLTs were able to deliver best practice care based on the NSF guidelines.

We found that early dysphasia intervention had further benefits in demonstrating clients' appropriateness for formal rehabilitation in the post-acute phase. For example, the rehabilitation team were able to witness early participation and progress in the acute setting, which in turn expedited clients' transfer to rehabilitation.

With these subjective positive outcomes associated with early dysphasia rehabilitation, we felt that it was worthwhile to compare our management of dysphasia at the RMH SCU with the management suggested in the literature. Attempts were made to provide therapy as early and as intensively as possible. The literature suggested intensive therapy, for at least two hours per week (Bhogal *et al.*, 2002; Robey, 1998). At the RMH SCU, only four sessions of approximately 20 minutes each were planned for each client per week. However, with other medical interventions and investigations one session was usually missed; thus most clients received approximately one hour of dysphasia therapy each week. Although it was not possible to deliver the amount of dysphasia therapy recommended by the literature, we were able nonetheless to significantly change our practice to better reflect the literature.

Reflections and key lessons

Some of the key lessons from our experience were the following points.

- When implementing a new or altered practice into clinical care, it is important to consider outcome measures to demonstrate change. In our case we felt overwhelmed by the thought of measuring the success of our project, particularly given stroke clients' tendency for spontaneous recovery. In hindsight, our evaluation of this project would have benefited from using outcome measures such as satisfaction surveys, as well as collecting process information such as the number of therapy hours each client received, and what therapy was implemented.

- It is imperative that clinicians engage with other members of their department and their broader team to develop strategies that will lead to the long-term uptake of an innovative way of delivering service. In our project we would have benefited from producing protocols and competency standards regarding therapy on the SCU, and including this information in our orientation package for SLTs who commenced on the unit.

This project led to benefits for clients, and led us to the realization that introducing an evidence-based approach to service planning does not need to be complicated or overwhelming. It is important to plan and communicate with a range of stakeholders. Maximizing available resources and considering local barriers and their solutions prior to commencing the project can lead to successful implementation of evidence-based service changes.

References

Bhogal, S., Teasell, R. and Speechley, M. (2002) Intensity of aphasia therapy, impact on recovery. *Stroke*, **34**, 987–993.

Enderby, P., Wood, V., Wade, D. and Hewer, R. (1987) Aphasia after stroke: a detailed study of recovery in the first 3 months. *International Rehabilitation Medicine*, **8**, 162–165.

Hartman, J. (1981) Measurement of early spontaneous recovery from aphasia in acute stroke. *Annals of Neurology*, **9**, 89–91.

Holland, A. and Fridriksson, J. (2001) Aphasia management during the early phases of recovery following stroke. *American Journal of Speech-Language Pathology*, **10** (1), 19–29.

Lalor, E. and Cranfield, E. (2004) Aphasia: a description of the incidence and management in the acute hospital setting. *Asia Pacific Journal of Speech, Language and Hearing*, **9**, 129–136.

National Stroke Foundation Australia (2007) Clinical guidelines for acute stroke management. Retrieved 9 October 2009 from http://www.strokefoundation.com.au/acute-clinical-guidelines-for-Acute-stroke-management.

Robey, R.R. (1998) A meta-analysis of clinical outcomes in the treatment of aphasia. *Journal of Speech, Language and Hearing Research*, **41** (1), 172–188.

Smithard, D., O'Neill, P., Park, C., *et al.* (1996) Complication and outcomes after acute stroke. Does dysphagia matter? *Stroke*, **27**, 1200–1204.

Weir, L. and Cadilhac, D.A. (2007) Managing a stroke unit: an example from Australia with an emphasis on nursing roles. *International Journal of Stroke*, **2** (3), 201–207.

26

Working with psychogenic dysphonia

Beth Higginbottom and Linda House

Speech and Language Therapists, Victoria Hospital, Blackpool, UK

The speech and language therapy (SLT) team in which we work is based in a large acute general hospital in the north-west of England. Our work involves management of an inpatient and outpatient caseload presenting with a wide variety of speech and language difficulties. In addition there are some smaller peripheral hospitals serving the wider community, which also provide inpatient and outpatient SLT services.

Our team is supported by a specialist SLT who has a designated role to promote research and evidence-based practice (a 'Research and Effectiveness' specialist role) and the whole team has a quarterly meeting focused on clinical development. This includes a journal club. These regular meetings enable the SLT team to continually develop knowledge and skills in as broad a range of subjects as possible.

Voice clients represent almost half of the outpatient caseload for the SLT team. We currently have no SLT specialist in voice, although it is recognized by the SLT team and the Ear, Nose and Throat (ENT) team that this would be needed for the future development of our provision to this client group. Unfortunately, several attempts to obtain funding to develop a specialist SLT voice service have been unsuccessful. In light of this, voice therapy is carried out by experienced therapists with generalist knowledge in the area of voice.

Standard practice for voice clients

The usual sequence of events for a person with a voice problem after referral by their family doctor is:

- attendance at the ENT clinic
- examination of the larynx by the otolaryngologist usually using flexible nasendoscopy
- dependent on the findings, the client may then be referred for assessment by the SLT team

- following SLT assessment, a course of voice therapy may be recommended and provided as appropriate.

Particularly complex voice clients may require further joint review with ENT and SLT, and this is arranged as needed.

The majority of voice clients respond to standard voice therapy, which by consensus generally includes: advice on care of the voice, relaxation, breath support for voice and vocal exercises. These would always be tailored to the needs of the client and would ideally take between four and six SLT sessions.

Working with clients with psychogenic dysphonia

There are a small number of dysphonic clients with muscle tension that remain resistant to such therapy. These clients tend to present with a strong psychogenic element which contributes significantly to the voice problem, and they often require a more holistic approach including counselling. The problem faced by the SLT is that these clients can then remain on the caseload or continually be re-referred for months or even years.

We determined a need to review the evidence to support management of these clients. We wanted to know, in adults with muscle tension dysphonia, with a strong psychogenic element, which is resistant to standard speech and language therapy treatment, what is the evidence for trying a completely different approach to standard therapy which helps the client achieve a better functional voice quality over a shorter period of therapy time?

Evaluating the evidence for non-standard therapy approaches

Research into the use of botulinum toxin treatment for spasmodic dysphonia was identified (Bhattacharyya and Tarsy, 2001). Botulinum treatment has been given to some of our clients with spasmodic dysphonia, and has also been used for at least one client with hyperkinetic dysphonia. Its use with other dysphonic clients, including those with muscle tension dysphonia, has not been supported by research evidence and therefore requires further evaluation.

Another option to treating the muscle tension directly would be to look at the causes of the psychogenic problem. This is discussed by Seifert E'Kollbrunner (2005) who suggests that additional counselling may be necessary for those where the psychosocial stress plays a greater role than the muscle tension in causing the dysphonia. Referral to counselling is always considered by the SLT team but is an addition to standard voice therapy rather than an alternative.

We became aware of another treatment to investigate when one of our long-term voice clients received ENT care at a neighbouring hospital. The client was seen at a joint voice clinic with the ENT Consultant and Voice SLT. Stroboscopy combined with rigid endoscopy was used to assess the client's vocal fold movement. During the course of this visit, the Voice SLT and ENT Consultant jointly recommended that the client would be appropriate for treatment with intravenous midazolam (a muscle relaxant). This was as a result of their recent joint research into the treatment of muscle tension dysphonia (Bhalla *et al.*, 2005). On discovery of such a treatment approach, we investigated the research behind it, and realized that it may be appropriate for other similar voice clients seen within our department.

The study supporting the use of midazolam (Bhalla *et al.*, 2005) was relatively small involving seven clients who had proved to be resistant to standard therapy over the previous two years. All seven clients had a diagnosis of muscle tension dysphonia with a strong psychogenic element. Midazolam was chosen for the study because it is a short acting benzodiazepine, which is rapidly metabolized by the liver, reducing the recovery time. The effect of the midazolam is to relax the client generally, but in particular their laryngeal muscles. The clients within the study were given the drug and then asked to produce voice whilst an audio recording was made. At this stage the voice was perceived as normal in most cases. Once the client had begun to recover from the effects of the drug (with the help of intravenous flumazenil), but was still in a relaxed state, they were then given 15 minutes of intensive therapy from the Voice SLT including kinaesthetic, auditory and visual feedback. In the seven resistant cases, six were found to require no further therapy for their voice one month after this intervention.

In order to gain further knowledge and to assess the evidence first hand, we attended the midazolam clinic (where Bhalla's research had been carried out) with the voice client who had been recommended for the treatment. The procedure was seen to be very quick and effective, with the voice client achieving near-normal voice immediately. The therapy given following administration of the drug was particularly effective due to the very relaxed state of the client and the intensity of the therapy; a level of which would not be possible during standard treatment.

Following the midazolam treatment this client's care was transferred back to our department for follow up therapy. We were able to implement some of the therapy strategies observed, but at a less intensive level. The client was able to achieve normal voice during therapy sessions, but was unable to maintain this in day-to-day situations. This is thought to be due to the significant and unresolved psychogenic issues, which are intractably part of this client's voice problem. Despite the client's inability to maintain the improvements gained through midazolam, it was recognized that this treatment would be suitable for some of our other long-term clients with therapy-resistant psychogenic/muscle tension dysphonia.

Implementing the evidence

From this experience we were able to identify a possible client (Lucy) from our own caseload for this intervention. As recommended in Bhalla's study (2005), Lucy exhibited muscle tension dysphonia together with a strong psychogenic element. She demonstrated a high level of anxiety and an abnormal pattern of laryngeal muscle use. She had received several episodes of standard therapy over a three-year period with no noticeable change to her voice.

Having identified the client we then went on to investigate the referral procedure for the treatment. We discovered that no one had previously been referred for this treatment from another SLT department; therefore there was no policy or procedure to follow. This resulted in a lengthy and complicated referral process, involving SLTs, two ENT consultants and the client's family doctor. The client was accepted for the treatment some months later.

Following our appraisal of the evidence, midazolam treatment was considered to be a potentially effective addition to standard therapy for a small number of voice clients. The evidence, and our personal experience with regard to this treatment were presented to the SLT team via a journal club at a regular team meeting. Further discussion lead to the team agreeing that this treatment should be made available to suitable clients for the following reasons:

- normal voice is restored (at least for a period of time)
- the procedure is quick and safe
- as the procedure is performed in the outpatient department, there is minimal inconvenience to the client
- there is a reduction in the amount of therapy required
- there are immediate functional and social benefits.

Although there are no lasting side effects of midazolam used in this way, some clients may be resistant to having any form of drug therapy, and this of course needs to be discussed prior to referral. As with any drug, midazolam can interact with other medication that the client may be taking, and in fact this was the case with Lucy discussed here. Lucy's midazolam treatment has had to be postponed for several months as she is taking pain relief medication unrelated to her voice problem. Therefore at the time of writing, the client still awaits midazolam treatment.

It was recognized by the SLT team that a procedure should be developed for referral for midazolam treatment. Creating a more straightforward referral process should encourage both SLTs and clients to access this treatment. We need to establish closer links with the SLT and ENT department providing the midazolam treatment in order to do this. It is presumed that there will be some financial implications in providing this treatment; for example would the SLT department be charged for referring clients? At this stage it is not known what limitations there may be. We need to ascertain how many of our clients would be accepted before we can include referral for midazolam treatment into our own management approach with this client group.

For the individual therapist, there may be training needs such as:

- learning how to identify suitable clients before extensive therapy is undertaken, and knowing at what point in therapy to consider making a referral
- providing effective follow-up therapy after midazolam treatment
- identifying other support that may be needed to maximize the benefits of the treatment.

Discussion, or a short training session with the SLT who conducted the research, may be possible to address this need, although it is currently not clear if this is available. It also needs to be acknowledged that once a therapist has invested a lot of therapy time and established a strong relationship with a client, it can be difficult to hand over the client to someone else. As therapists, we need to be able to objectively consider the evidence for best practice and act upon this accordingly.

Ideally, midazolam treatment would be available within our SLT department. This would require in-depth training for both a lead SLT and an ENT Consultant. To our knowledge, the researchers have not promoted a training programme for the procedure although it may be possible to approach them directly regarding this. As previously mentioned, having no voice specialist SLT, and limited liaison with ENT, it will be difficult to offer this form of treatment ourselves. We felt that it should only be offered by therapists with appropriate knowledge and experience, who have developed this treatment with the co-operation and guidance of their ENT department.

Reflections

Despite the barriers and the difficulties we may have in implementing the changes suggested by the evidence, it is felt that the learning experience has been positive and worthwhile, and will lead to changes in our practice with these clients. Now that this knowledge is available to our department we can use it as far as is possible by hopefully developing more formal links between our neighbouring SLT/ ENT department and ourselves.

This experience has highlighted that to fully implement a new treatment, such as the use of midazolam, requires a specialist SLT to lead the development. In addition, as this evidence was discovered almost by chance, there appears to be a need for increased transparency and communication between members of our profession and more publicity for important new innovations.

Acknowledgements

With thanks to Jane Wallis (SLT) and Mr de Carpentier (ENT Consultant) for accepting our voice clients into their continuing research programme.

References

Bhalla, R.K., Wallis, J., Kaushik, V. and de Carpentier, J.P. (2005) How we do it: adjunctive intravenous midazolam: diagnosis and treatment of therapy-resistant muscle tension dysphonia. *Clinical Otolaryngology*, **30**, 364–383.

Bhattacharyya, N. and Tarsy, D. (2001) Impact on quality of life of botulinum toxin treatments for spasmodic dysphonia and oromandibular dystonia. *Archives of Otolaryngology Head and Neck Surgery*, **127**, 389–392.

Seifert E' Kollbrunner, J. (2005) Stress and distress in non-organic voice disorder. *Swiss Medical Weekly*, **135** (27–28), 387–397.

27

Implementation of a free fluid protocol in an aged care facility

Amanda Scott[1] and Leora Benjamin[2]

[1]Senior Speech Pathologist, The Alfred Hospital, Melbourne, Australia
[2]Speech Pathologist, Caulfield General Medical Centre, Melbourne, Australia

This chapter describes the implementation of a free fluid protocol (FFP) for dysphagic residents in a 45-bed aged care facility. The authors are speech and language therapists (SLTs) with extensive experience in dysphagia research and management in acute, rehabilitation and palliative care settings. They also have a keen interest in aged care. The project described in this chapter was undertaken in a residential aged-care facility in Melbourne, Australia.

SLTs routinely recommend that people with dysphagia have thickened fluids to prevent or reduce the risk of aspiration. Aspiration, due to impaired airway protection during swallowing, is a recognized risk factor for developing pneumonia. Because thickened fluids move more slowly through the pharynx compared to thin fluids, impaired pharyngeal and laryngeal muscles have more time to respond as supported by observations made during videofluoroscopic assessments of swallowing by Scott (1999).

Although thickened fluids are thought to address the safety aspect of fluid intake several other factors need to be considered. Residents in aged care facilities who have chronically impaired swallowing may have thickened fluids recommended as part of SLT management, but in our experience, they frequently complain that they do not quench their thirst and are 'claggy' in the mouth. The limited range of thickened fluids usually available (i.e. fruit juices and milk drinks) are not the type of drinks residents want to have in large amounts. These factors contribute to reduced fluid intake and an increased risk of dehydration for residents having thickened fluids. Denial of favourite drinks, such as tea or water, has a negative impact on the quality of life. Consequently, there is often poor compliance with the recommendation of 'thickened fluids only' in residential aged care settings. The observation that residents with dysphagia who have thin fluid do not always develop pneumonia (Hartlage and Panther, 1992) highlights the need to investigate this further.

Examining the evidence for dysphagia management

We decided to examine the safety of providing thin fluids to dysphagic residents. As this represented a departure from accepted SLT practice, we examined the evidence pertaining to thickened fluids to see if studies had identified their benefits and/or problems. We also reviewed the literature for direct links between aspiration pneumonia and thin fluids. Finally, we looked at literature related to dehydration because we were concerned that residents having thickened fluids had low fluid intake. We used the electronic databases CINAHL and Medline, as well as a librarian-assisted search, dividing papers between the authors to summarize the relevant information.

The efficacy of thickened fluids

The first aspect of the project was to examine the efficacy of thickened fluid. The findings are inconclusive, and often difficult to decipher, as dysphagia management programs that have been assessed in the literature include multiple aspects, and not just the use of thickened fluids (e.g. Doggett *et al.*, 2001). Other studies reported modifications of both food and fluid, making it difficult to know the contribution of the fluid consistency to the reported rate of aspiration (e.g. Groher, 1987). A single randomized, controlled trial (RCT) was identified that examined the effects of unlimited intake of water in patients with identified aspiration (Garon *et al*, 1997). This study monitored two groups of ten stroke patients, randomized to receive either free water or thickened fluids. At the end of a twelve month period no one in either group had developed pneumonia, dehydration or any other related medical complication. However, the free water protocol group had higher levels of satisfaction, with only one in the thickened fluid group indicating that they were happy with the thickened fluids. This study lends support to the practice of giving free fluid to dysphagic patients. There have been some reports on negative consequences of fluids thickened using guar gum. Risks include bowel impaction, severe constipation and gastric reflux (Victorian Department of Human Services, 2006).

Aspiration pneumonia

The causes of pneumonia are more complex than aspiration of ingested material associated with dysphagia. Accurate diagnosis of aspiration pneumonia can be difficult. There are no specific tests with diagnosis usually based on clinical observations. Various papers have identified other factors associated with the development of aspiration pneumonia, including:

- nasogastric tubes, tracheostomy tubes, or poor oral health, as these are associated with pathogenic bacteria (Johnson and Hirsch, 2003; Kikawada *et al.*, 2005; Terpenning *et al.*, 2001);
- reduced ability to effectively clear material from the lungs associated with chronic obstruction pulmonary disease, congestive cardiac failure, bronchiectasis and bronchial obstruction (Johnson and Hirsch, 2003), and
- patient factors, such as generalized weakness and immobility, reduced level of consciousness, multiple medications, or neurogenic diagnosis (Langmore *et al.*, 1998).

The literature suggested that the type of material that is aspirated may be particularly important. For example Johnson and Hirsch (2003) argued that particulate material is more difficult to expectorate than liquid, and therefore may present an increased risk. Holas *et al.* (1994) also suggested that thickened fluid is more difficult to expectorate than thin fluid, which was of particular interest to our review.

Dehydration

The evidence suggested that dehydration is the most common fluid and electrolyte problem in the elderly. It is associated with a range of medical problems including increased risk of stroke recurrence (Burger *et al.*, 2001), and increased susceptibility to urinary tract infections, pneumonia, renal failure and decubitus ulcers (Kelly *et al.*, 2004). A recent study by Robbins *et al.* (2008) showed that patients having thickened fluid had an increased incidence of dehydration (6% compared to 2%). Other studies identified that patients given thickened fluids had inadequate fluid intakes (Finestone *et al.*, 2001; Whelan, 2001). Philip and Greenwood (2000) suggested that patients on thickened fluids were offered fewer drinks than those on free fluids, while Chidester and Spangler (2001) reported that elderly residents receive adequate fluids on meal trays but that their actual intake is insufficient, specifically when thickened fluids are given.

Implementation of the evidence in clinical practice

Following our review of the current evidence the SLT team decided to introduce a free fluid protocol (FFP). This was approved by the hospital Clinical Practice Committee and the nursing home residents' doctors were provided with written information about the project. The FFP was adapted from the free water protocol, developed at the Frazier Rehabilitation Center, in the USA (Panther, 2005). The Frazier protocol was reported to have been successfully used since 1984, and to fit the needs of the current nursing home. The basic protocol is outlined in Box 27.1.

We collected data over a ten month period, in order to evaluate the FFP in our setting, and to contribute to the evidence in this area.

Evaluation of the FFP for residents

Residents participating in the trial of the FFP were first assessed by the SLTs. Twenty-six residents were given free fluid over a ten month period. These people (N = 16 male and N = 10 female) had an average age of 78 years (range 45–95 years) and had a range of conditions typical of residents found in aged care set-

---

Box 27.1   The free fluid protocol

Supervised sips of water, tea and coffee are allowed:

- between meals only, not with food or medications
- half an hour after food
- only when sitting upright
- strict oral care after eating

tings, including dementia, neurological impairment (including stroke), cardiac disease, respiratory disease, and renal disease. SLTs were asked to record their decision-making for each resident allowed the free fluids in this trial. It was found that the resident instigated the decision in 38% of cases, either by a direct request, or by actively refusing to have thickened fluids. In the remaining 16 cases, the decision was instigated following discussions between staff and family members, and rationales included concern about the unappealing nature of thickened fluid, concern about fluid intake, or observation that the resident was taking free fluid inappropriately, such as drinking directly from a tap or vase.

In order to evaluate the safety of the protocol the participants' health was monitored bi-monthly for eight months. There were no clear negative changes in their health that could be directly related to the FFP. No instances of pneumonia occurred, and there were no new episodes of acute illness in the residents. There were three deaths, two relating to pre-existing medical conditions and one relating to aspiration of vomit. Those with pre-existing respiratory symptoms continued to evidence these problems without change.

Reflections on the implementation of the FFP

Free fluid practices are in place at an informal level in many aged care settings. The findings of our small-scale evaluation are consistent with the outcomes of the small RCT conducted by Garon et al. (1997), demonstrating that there is a continued need for ongoing data to improve our understanding of the management of dysphagia. Both safety and quality of life need to be considered.

Although there are few definitive studies in this area, the literature had some clear messages that guided our decision making: that free fluid does not appear to increase the risk of pneumonia (Garon et al., 1997), that aspiration pneumonia is related to many factors including the type of fluid (Holas et al., 1994; Johnson and Hirsch, 2003) and that residents on thickened fluids were at increased risk of dehydration because of decreased fluid intake (Finestone et al., 2001; Robbins et al., 2008; Whelan, 2001). Weighing up this evidence, we decided to implement the policy. Our evaluation showed that it was used safely, and we continue to closely monitor patients with dysphagic symptoms who are given free fluids. The FFP was easily adopted by staff in this facility, perhaps because they had already observed some of the problems with thickened fluids which have also been shown in the literature (e.g. reduced fluid intake in residents). The commitment of management, who saw the importance of the FFP and were also supportive of the additional benefits in terms of oral health training that were needed, was also essential to the success of this project. We have also received many enquiries about the project from other SLTs in Australia, suggesting that the question of giving free water is of interest in other facilities. The project was highly commended in the 2006 Victorian Public Healthcare Awards.

References

Burger, S.G., Kayser-Jones, J. and Bell, J.P. (2001) Food for thought: Preventing/treating malnutrition and dehydration. *Contemporary Long-Term Care*, **24** (4), 24–28.

Chidester, J.C. and Spangler, A.A. (2001) Fluid intake in the institutionalized elderly. *Journal of the American Dietetic Association*, **97** (1).

Doggett, D.L., Tappe, K.L., Mitchell, M.D., Chapell, R., Coates, V. and Turkelson, C.M. (2001) Prevention of pneumonia in elderly stroke patients by systematic diagnosis and treatment of dysphagia: An evidence-based comprehensive analysis of the literature. *Dysphagia*, **16**, 279–295.

Finestone, H.M., Foley, N.C., Woodbury, M.G. and Greene-Finestone, L. (2001) Quantifying fluid intake in dysphagic stroke patients: A preliminary comparison of oral and nonoral strategies. *Archives of Physical Medicine and Rehabilitation*, **82** (12), 1744–1746.

Garon, B., Engle, M. and Ormiston, C. (1997) A randomized control study to determine the effects of unlimited oral intake of water in patients with identified aspiration. *Journal of Neurological Rehabilitation*, **11**, 139–148.

Groher, M.E. (1987) Bolus management and aspiration pneumonia in patients with pseudobulbar dysphagia. *Dysphagia*, **1** (4), 215–216.

Hartlage, C. and Panther, K. (1992) New directions in dysphagia. *Network Newsletter*, **2** (4), 2–3.

Holas, M.A., DePippo, K.L. and Reding, M.J. (1994) Aspiration and relative risk of medical complications following stroke. *Archives of Neurology*, **51**, 1051–1053.

Johnson, J.L. and Hirsch, C.S. (2003) Aspiration pneumonia: recognising and managing a potentially growing disorder [electronic version]. *Postgraduate Medicine Online*, **11**, 1–13 from http://www.postgradmed.com.

Kelly, J., Hunt, B.J., Lewis, R.R., *et al.* (2004) Dehydration and venous thromboembolism after acute stroke. *Quarterly Journal of Medicine*, **97** (5), 293–296.

Kikawada, M., Iwamoto, T. and Takasaki, M. (2005) Aspiration and infection in the elderly: Epidemiology, diagnosis and management. *Drugs and Ageing*, **22** (2), 115–130.

Langmore, S.E., Terpenning, M.S., Schork, A., *et al.* (1998). Predictors of aspiration pneumonia: How important is dysphagia. *Dysphagia*, **13**, 69–81.

Panther, K. (2005) Free Water Protocol, The Frazier Rehabilitation Center. Retrieved 11 October 2009, from http://www.jhsmh.org/carecenters/re_sp_waterpro.asp

Philip, C. and Greenwood, K. (2000) Nutrient contribution of infant cereals used as fluid thickening agents in diets fed to the elderly. *Journal of the American Dietetic Association*, **100** (5), 549–554.

Robbins, J., Gensler, G., Hind, J., *et al.* (2008) Comparison of two interventions for liquid aspiration on pneumonia incidence. *Annals of Internal Medicine*, **148** (7), 209–518.

Scott, A. (1999) The development of a scale to assess swallowing function in motor neurone disease using videofluoroscopic techniques. Unpublished PhD, La Trobe University, Melbourne, Australia.

Terpenning, M.S., Taylor, G.W., Lopatin, D.E., Kinder Kerr, C., iza Dominguez, L. and Loesche, W.J. (2001) Aspiration pneumonia: Dental and oral risk factors in an older veteran population. *Journal of the American Geriatrics Society*, **49** (5), 557–563.

Victorian Department of Human Services (2006) Drinking and fluids – maintaining hydration (Well for Life Help Sheet No. 14) [electronic version]. Retrieved 9 May 2009 from http://www.health.vic.gov.au/agedcare/publications/wellforlife/wellforlife_hs14.pdf.

Whelan, K. (2001) Inadequate fluid intakes in dysphagic acute stroke. *Clinical Nutrition*, **20** (5), 423–428.

28

Prosody intervention for children

Christina Samuelsson

Senior lecturer, Department of Clinical and Experimental Medicine/Logopedics, Faculty of Health Sciences, Linköping University, Sweden

Prosody carries a lot of information relevant for the understanding of spoken messages. In addition, prosody plays an important role in signalling attitudes and emotions. Prosody can be described as the rhythmic, dynamic and melodic features of language. There is no direct correspondence between perceptual judgements of prosody and instrumental measures (Hargrove and McGarr, 1994). The acoustic–phonetic properties related to prosody are duration, intensity and pitch. Intonation is perhaps the most salient prosodic feature and thereby much involved in the perception of prosody. Swedish has a complicated prosodic system, compared to English and a large proportion of Swedish children with language impairment (LI) have prosodic problems to some extent. In Swedish, there are contrasts of vowel quantity and word stress as well as of tonal word accents. There are a few hundred minimal pairs distinguished by tonal word accent alone (Elert, 1966). A number of minimal pairs can be found where the placement of stress is distinctive. However, the placement of stress is not the only difference between these words since the quality of both consonants and vowels is affected by stress (Cruttenden, 1997; Bruce, 1998).

Prosody has previously not been the focus of research in Swedish children with LI, but in 2004 I completed my dissertation on this topic. Clinically, prosodic problems often are noted by speech and language therapists (SLTs), but they report that they are not very confident in either assessing prosody or intervening with it. There are also not many descriptions in the literature of prosody intervention, which means that clinicians must rely on their overall linguistic and therapeutic knowledge when designing intervention for prosodic problems.

The clinical problem

A four-year-old boy (Max) presented to a local SLT clinic with phonological language impairment and difficulties with lexical prosody at the phrase and discourse level. The clinician had a question about Max's prosody, which she felt needed further investigation. She contacted me at Linköping University, as I have previously published and spoken about prosodic problems.

I undertook a literature review to understand the clinical problem. The evidence in this area is not very extensive, and most of it is presented here. Within the scope of a research project, a comprehensive assessment procedure to capture Swedish prosodic features at word, phrase and discourse level had been developed (Samuelsson et al., 2003). In order to elicit the target structures, the test uses different elicitation strategies, such as direct questions, sentence completion, modelling, video narration and formalized conversational questions. The assessment procedure has been used to estimate the prevalence of prosodic problems in Swedish children with LI and also to characterize these problems. It was found that 41% of children with severe LI, recruited from local Language Units, had prosodic problems to some extent (Samuelsson et al., 2003). In another study, children with prosodic problems were compared to children with typical language (TL) development and it was found that children with LI in combination with prosodic problems performed significantly worse than children with TL at all levels of the assessment procedure (Samuelsson and Nettelbladt, 2004). It was also shown that prosodic problems can be grouped into subcategories, where 33% of the children with LI had prosodic problems mainly at word level, 42% had prosodic problems at both word and phrase level and 17% were identified as having prosodic problems mainly at discourse level.

The evidence suggested that prosodic problems could exist at the word, phrase and discourse level, and thus, thorough assessment was needed in all of these areas. Additionally, both production and perception of prosody should be assessed at each level. Language intervention can be defined as deliberate efforts by professionals and families to help children with LI strengthen their linguistic ability (Leonard, 1998). Today, intervention for children with LI most often has a child-centred, dialogical perspective. Intervention can focus on perception, production or both, depending on the nature and severity of the impairment (Nettelbladt et al., 2008). Ideally, a model of intervention should fit the interests and the personality of the child, focus on crucial aspects of speech and language and be suited to the child's communication needs. Specific to prosodic problems, the evidence suggested that, even though prosody is a complex and multifaceted entity, prosody intervention can benefit from adopting a discrete approach. That is, prosody is subdivided into manageable units called prosodic components, such as tempo, intonation, stress and rhythm (Hargrove and McGarr, 1994).

Implementing the evidence for management of prosodic problems

An assessment and intervention programme was designed on the basis of existing evidence. A multiple baseline single-subject design (Hegde, 1987) was used to evaluate the intervention. Max's prosody was assessed repeatedly (three times during a period of nine weeks), using the previously described assessment tool. In addition, assessment was also made of other linguistic skills, such as grammatical skills and language comprehension. The assessment showed that Max had problems with prosodic production at word level (where he scored 68% correct), at phrase level (80% correct) and at discourse level (where his problems were scored as moderately deviant on a three-level categorical scale). His perception of prosodic contrasts was considerably better than his production. His prosodic problems were shown to be stable across observations, which means that they provide contrast to treatment effects, since they did not recover spontaneously during the assessment period of nine weeks. As regards grammatical abilities and language comprehension, Max achieved results at age level.

The intervention was designed by the researcher and the clinician in collaboration but carried out exclusively by the clinician. The basic goal was to improve Max's prosodic abilities at word, phrase and discourse levels; intermediate goals were to increase his ability to produce prosodic contrasts at all levels; specific goals were formulated at each level. The main focus was on word level and different intonation and stress patterns were practised both perceptually and by production. Since Max's perception was better than his production he was assumed to benefit from exercises where he could rely on his perceptual skills. Tonal word accents and early versus late stress was practised using minimal pairs with two pictures of, for example, /kàfɛ/ – /kafé:/ = 'coffee' – 'café' or /tómtɛn/ – /tòmtɛn/ = 'the garden' – 'Santa Claus' (see Figure 28.1).

Concerning phrasal prosody, phrasal stress and intonation was practised by means of imitation, both of real phrases and of nonsense phrases where both stress and intonation were varied. The structures that were practised, both real and nonsense, were not the same as those that are part of the assessment procedure. Work on discourse prosody was carried out by means of recording and listening together with Max, which made him more aware of the importance of prosodic features. In this part of the intervention the Max's perceptual skills were encouraged. The intervention comprised six sessions of one hour each. Alongside the work at the clinic, the parents were instructed to work on prosody at both word and phrase level at home. Working material, such as card games and work sheets, were sent home.

The intervention was evaluated with the assessment procedure used before intervention. Evaluations were made right at the end of the intervention period and again three months later. The results indicate that the intervention was effective and Max showed improved prosodic skills at both word and phrase level. Perceptual evaluation also revealed slight improvement at discourse level. In an interview with the parent it was also found that Max found the intervention pleasant and his compliance was good. The assessment three months later also indicates that the results are stable; Max has even continued to improve during this post-intervention period.

Reflections

Due to the limitations of the literature, we designed an assessment and intervention program that was based on existing evidence, but also added to the evidence using a single-subject study. Evaluation of new intervention strategies is very well suited for small research projects such as this, and in this work the close collaboration between clinician and researcher has been very fruitful.

The good result of the intervention probably has multiple explanations. First, the timing of the intervention was good, Max was receptive and motivated and

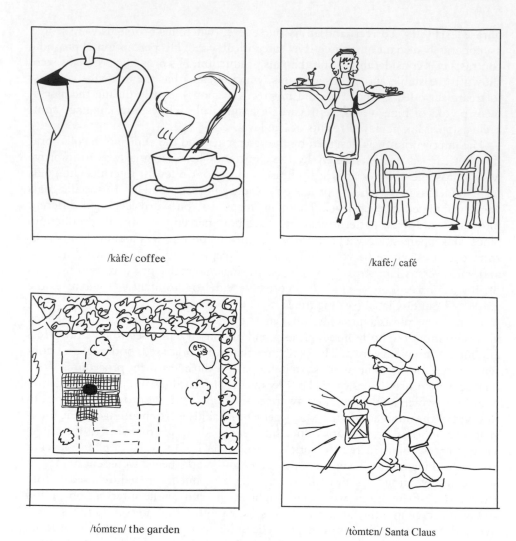

/kàfɛ/ coffee

/kafé:/ café

/tómtɛn/ the garden

/tòmtɛn/ Santa Claus

Figure 28.1 Pictures from the training material.

his parents had opportunities to work with him at home. Good timing is essential for intervention, but it is very hard to estimate when the timing is optimal. Second, the assessment of Max's prosodic problems was made very thoroughly and in accordance with previous research on Swedish children with LI. In terms of evidence based practice (EBP), the assessment relates to the first of the recommended steps in an EBP approach, which is referred to as 'formulating the clinical question' (McCauly and Fey, 2006; McCauly and Hargrove, 2004). A thorough assessment is needed both in order to determine problem areas and to identify aspects of the prosodic system that are intact and that may be available for compensatory strategies (Hargrove and McGarr, 1994). The assessment in the present implementation project comprised both perceptual and productive prosody at word, phrase and discourse level and the relative strength of Max's prosodic perception abilities were used in intervention. Thirdly, the intervention was highly individualized and it was designed in accordance with research findings on prosodic development. Traditionally, prosodic intervention approaches tend to be problem rather than model driven and clinicians usually select goals without reference to prosody as a whole (Hargrove and McGarr, 1994). In the present project, ordering objectives in relation to the assessment procedure probably contributed to good intervention results. Finally, the close co-operation between the researcher and the clinician in the present project made it possible to carry out the intervention near the patient. The clinician's knowledge about Max and his family also contributed to make the intervention tailor-made.

In order to make speech and language therapy increasingly evidence based, there is a need for more published evidence of the effectiveness of speech and language intervention. The single-subject design as described in the present chapter is a very useful way of documenting and describing outcomes of intervention. It is also important to base and design implementation projects on existing research, since this is a very fruitful way of adding up knowledge on different clinical problems.

Acknowledgements

First and foremost, I would like to express my gratitude to Max, and his mother for bringing him every week. I would also like to thank the collaborating clinician for her great interest in the study, valuable comments and of course for carrying out the intervention.

References

Bruce, G. (1998). *General and Swedish prosody* [Swedish]. Dept. of Linguistics, Lund University.

Cruttenden, A. (1997) *Intonation*. New York: University Press.

Elert, C.-C. (1966) *General and Swedish Phonetics* [in Swedish]. Stockholm: Almqvist and Wiksell Förlag AB.

Hargrove, P. and McGarr, N. (1994) *Prosody Management of Communication Disorders*. San Diego: Singular.

Hegde, M.N. (1987) *Clinical Research in Communicative Disorders. Principles and Strategies*. Austin, TX: Pro-Ed.

Leonard, L.B. (1998) *Children with Specific Language Impairment*. Cambridge, MA: MIT Press.

McCauly, R.J. and Fey, M.E. (2006) *Treatment of Language Disorders in Children*. Baltimore: Paul H. Brooks Publishing Co.

McCauly, R.J. and Hargrove, P. (2004) A clinician's introduction to systematic reviews in communication disorders: The course review paper with muscle. *Contemporary Issues in Communication Science and Disorders*, 31, 173–181.

Nettelbladt, U., Samuelsson, C., Sahlén, B. and Hansson, K. (2008) Language impairment in children without other disabilities [in Swedish]. In L. Hartelius, U. Nettelbladt and B. Hammarberg (eds), *Logopedi*. Lund: Studentlitteratur, pp. 139–147.

Samuelsson, C. and Nettelbladt, U. (2004) Prosodic problems in Swedish children with language impairment: towards a classification of subgroups. *International Journal of Language and Communication Disorders*, **39** (3), 325–344.

Samuelsson, C., Scocco, C. and Nettelbladt, U. (2003) Towards assessment of prosodic abilities in Swedish children with language impairment. *Logopedics Phoniatrics Vocology*, **28**, 156–166.

29 Supporting evidence-based practice for students on placement: making management decisions for clients with Down Syndrome

Ruth Miller

Speech and Language Therapist, Manchester Primary Care Trust, UK

I am a speech and language therapist (SLT) working in paediatrics and specializing in developing the communication skills of children with severe and profound learning difficulties. I work in the context of a school designated as a National Specialist College for Special Educational Needs, which specializes in cognition and learning and places a strong emphasis on collaborative working with a range of partners. The College caters for pupils aged from 11 to 19 years with severe or profound complex and persistent learning difficulties.

In this school context, intervention takes a variety of forms, including individual sessions, group work and consultative advice to teachers. In our service, SLT students are allocated on placement each year from one of two universities in the city. Whilst students on placement can be at any stage of their training, those at an earlier stage can struggle to get to grips both with the normal processes of language development and their application to adolescents with learning difficulties. This chapter describes the journey for two students who were in their second year of training, and for whom a supported approach to developing a clinical question, accessing the evidence, and applying the evidence, was used. This approach facilitated their own clinical learning, and allowed an evidence-based approach to intervention for two clients with Down Syndrome (DS).

Supporting students to identify the clinical question

Each SLT student was assigned a client with DS to work with over the course of their placement, which would entail one session per week over a period of eight weeks. These were the first clients the students had ever worked with in the course of their training. Both of these clients, Liam and Daniel, were males aged sixteen years. Each had good lexical abilities and functional pragmatic skills, but like many adolescents with DS used very short, basic subject–verb, subject–verb–object, subject–verb–adverb sentence structure with little expansion at phrase level and little morphological marking. They each had additional difficulties, namely phonological issues and, for Daniel, fluency issues, which impeded intelligibility to some extent. Both had some knowledge and use of approximately 20–30 signs from the 'Communication Link' sign vocabulary that was developed at Beverley School for Deaf Children (1998) in Middlesbrough, UK.

In order to formulate their clinical questions the SLT students first observed the SLT working with the clients and then spent time getting to know the clients in informal conversation, following this with a series of simple formal assessments. They were encouraged to record their findings and to begin to discuss their observations. Both students were struck by the wide range of the boys' communication difficulties on a number of levels and were keen to explore possible strategies for intervention. At the same time they needed to develop their as yet limited knowledge of DS and revisit and apply their previous learning of normal language development. Our discussions at this point then became wider ranging and encompassed issues relating to the following points.

- *The clients themselves.* For example, would the clients be able to move beyond their basic language level and would it be worth setting up an intervention programme to try to develop their language further? Would we be better leaving it to 'natural' processes, or was there evidence that language would remain at a basic level whatever we did? Should we continue to develop signing in these pupils, given that they had some comprehension and expressive language, and if so, what would be our justification for this?
- *Our knowledge about DS.* For example, we considered what we knew about how language and communication develop in adolescents with DS and what were the proven approaches and strategies for adolescents with DS.
- *The practicalities of the clients' learning environment.* This was relevant in terms of encouraging school staff to follow guidance relating to these clients. For example, staff may express reservations about signing on the basis that they believe it might encourage the clients to sign rather than to develop their spoken language. We needed to consider whether there would be certain preferences in the school for certain approaches (e.g. group work).
- *The SLT students' learning experience.* For example, we questioned what the learning outcomes for the students should be as a result of working with these two clients (e.g. increased knowledge of language development and of DS, proficiency in the practical management of the clinical situation, ability to apply their theoretical knowledge to experience, and so on).

The students were then encouraged to summarize and reformulate their general discussion questions into a smaller number of clear clinical questions (Box 29.1).

Box 29.1 Clinical questions formulated on the basis of student observations and discussions

1. Is there evidence for continued language development in clients with DS in the late teenage years?
2. If so, which language approaches or strategies have proven benefit with clients of this age?
3. Is there evidence for benefits of encouraging/teaching signing?

This was used to enable us to maintain a more specific focus with which to approach the literature, to formulate simple and clear objectives for our sessions with the clients, and to provide a clear rationale for teaching staff concerning our intervention with the clients.

Consulting the evidence for working with adolescents with DS

We consulted Rondal and Buckley's (2003) book on *Speech and Language Intervention in Down Syndrome*. This book has a focus on the appraisal of evidence for intervention for both adults and children with DS. It covers a wide range of topics relevant to speech and language therapy intervention from a number of experts in the field who have summarized and appraised the wider literature and who are able to give pointers for further exploration. The book was one known to the students in name, and used and recommended by other SLTs in the department working with infants and children with DS. For students whose skills in searching the literature and critical appraisal are at an early stage, such texts can be a good starting point or scaffold for development of these skills and can present a less daunting prospect than tackling from the outset the mountain of literature available of relevance to this field.

The chapter on 'Continued language intervention with adolescents and adults with Down Syndrome' by Christine Jenkins (2003) was particularly helpful to our questions about working with 16-year-old clients. Jenkins describes the hypotheses of the 'critical period' and the 'syntactic ceiling', proposed and researched by previous authors (Lenneberg, 1967; Fowler, 1990), suggesting a limited potential for language development in clients with DS beyond childhood and beyond simple structures. She then presents evidence which challenges these hypotheses (Leddy and Gill, 1999; Jenkins, 2001) and examples from the literature of successful interventions with teenagers and young adults in this client group, eg visual strategies (including signing and reading) and structured language teaching (Bray and Woolnough, 1988; Leddy and Gill, 1999).

As a result of her appraisal of the literature, the strategies recommended by Jenkins (2003) when working with adolescents with DS include:

- building on strengths in the visual domain, particularly signing and reading
- using structured language programmes to expand language use
- incorporating programmes into group work to encourage generalization
- developing strategies to repair communication breakdown.

Thus, in answer to our three questions, the literature, as summarized by Jenkins (2003), suggested that:

- language development could be improved in these clients
- there was evidence for some specific approaches with this client group (using visual skills, group work)
- given the recommendation to build on visual skills, there were likely to be benefits to encouraging signing with these clients.

In addition to this, the students could recognize that they needed to revisit their own learning on areas of language development, for example, morphosyntactic development (e.g. Rondal, 2003).

Developing evidence-based language programmes

Armed with the knowledge gained during this process, the SLT students then wrote structured language programmes for their respective clients, aiming to develop comprehension and expression by building up phrases (e.g. incorporating qualifiers like colour or size adjectives into noun phrases, or prepositions and articles into adverbial phrases), and incorporating both signing and use of pictures, symbols and written words. They were supported by the SLT and each other to implement these programmes with both clients. We also looked at the potential for the clients to be included in work in language groups, an approach which is preferred by the school as it provides greater opportunity for collaborative working between teachers and SLTs. There was also a recommendation from the evidence that showed a need to support generalization. Communication repair skills were targeted in language sessions, through deliberately setting up sabotage situations in their individual work, for example, pretending we had not understood, and reassuring them that it was acceptable to say, 'No…' and then use sign to expand their meaning.

Over the course of the students' placement, the two clients made steady progress, notably in the expansion of their language at phrase level. This was evidenced in small improvements in their scores on the formal tests, although the fact that these tests are not specifically developed for adolescents with learning difficulties meant that the gains made by the clients seemed limited. More significant in evidencing progress were the students' recorded incidence of the clients' target phrases and use of signing during sessions, and, in the wider context, the spontaneous comments of teaching staff at school on the improvements in the expressive language use of Liam (although less so in the case of Daniel, whose fluency and intelligibility were more severely impaired).

Reflections on this experience

As a busy clinician, taking on student placements can be difficult, particularly when they are at an early level in their training and require a high amount of support. It can seem like an impossible task to also expect them to be reviewing and incorporating learning from research evidence into their clinical practice. However, supporting students can serve to remind clinicians of the essential need for '… the integration of best research evidence with clinical expertise and patient values' (Sackett et al., 1997, p. 1) and encourage the clinician to be more explicit about their own decision-making process with clients in order to support students to develop these skills.

With appropriate support and scaffolding, we have found that even students on their first clinical placement are able to grasp the need to base their management decisions on research evidence as well as their clinical findings and assessment of clients' preferences. They are also able to start to develop literature searching and critical appraisal skills which they will further hone as they progress in their training.

The students in this case were supported to formulate useful and appropriate clinical questions. These were driven by a need to summarize and simplify the wide range of issues arising from their experience (e.g. observation and assessment) of the clients, as well as the need to formulate clear, realistic objectives for the clients. In our experience, students can find it very difficult to formulate simple, focussed objectives and session plans and to support these with a clear evidence-based rationale, which guides and supports the intervention process with the client.

Given the vast quantity of literature in books and journals on communication in DS, the challenge for busy clinicians and students is to select the most accessible evidence and, further, to be able to critically appraise the evidence rather than simply accept it on face value. Identifying an appropriate source of pre-appraised literature – the text by Rondal and Buckley (2003) – was an important strategy for supporting the students in this case. Rather than sending them straight to a wide range of journal articles, we relied primarily on Jenkins (2003), who summarizes the evidence for the questions that the students had formulated. Other sources that might be useful for students include:

- evidence-based clinical guidelines
- journal articles reporting systematic reviews of the area
- journals that publish critical appraisals of papers (e.g. *Evidence-Based Communication Assessment and Intervention*, published by Psychology Press).

In all these sources, the evidence has been appraised and summarized, and students can learn the principles of EBP without being reliant on their own limited critical appraisal skills. Nevertheless, the challenge for both students and qualified clinicians in their ongoing clinical development is to continue to develop their critical appraisal skills and to integrate the research findings into their management of specific cases, and this should be the understanding on which sources of pre-appraised literature are consulted.

In terms of the wider benefits of this experience, the SLT students themselves felt that consulting the evidence had led to a sense of confidence in making appropriate intervention decisions and developing structured language programmes, particularly at such an early stage in their training when faced with a specialist situation. Both the students and I felt it had been a helpful step away from a reliance on received teaching and directed reading towards a greater independence in searching, appraising and applying the literature to a specific clinical case. This in turn had paved the way for their ongoing work in future placements and in their future clinical careers.

In addition to these outcomes for the students, there were also significant outcomes for other staff at the school. Certain teaching and support staff working with the two clients on a day to day basis were keen to take on board some of the issues identified by our reading of the literature. For example, they felt encouraged to use signing with pupils with a range of communication abilities, not just those with very limited verbal expression. The evidence also supported the need for group work for language development; this is now generally preferred throughout the school, and is arguably the best context in which to practise social communication and emerging language skills. The SLT and teaching staff and are now developing some packages for different facets of communication (attention and listening; expanding sentence use; social interaction skills; use of symbols and pictures to support communication development) for teachers' use in these groups.

References

Beverley School for Deaf Children (1998) *Communication Link: A dictionary of signs* (3rd edn). Middlesbrough, UK: Cleveland Sign Resource Project.

Bray, M. and Woolnough, L. (1988) The language skills of children with Down's syndrome aged 12–16 years. *Child Language Teaching and Therapy*, 4 (3), 311–324.

Fowler, A. (1990) Language abilities in children with Down syndrome: Evidence for a specific syntactic delay. In D. Ciccetti and M. Beeghly (eds), *Children in Down Syndrome: A Developmental Perspective*. New York: Cambridge University Press, pp. 302–328.

Jenkins, C. (2001) Adults with Down syndrome: an investigation of the effect of reading on language skills. Unpublished PhD thesis. University of Portsmouth, Portsmouth.

Jenkins, C. (2003) Continued language intervention with adolescents and adults with Down syndrome. In J.A. Rondal and S. Buckley (eds), *Speech and Language Intervention in Down Syndrome*. London: Whurr, pp. 154–165.

Leddy, M. and Gill, G. (1999) Enhancing the speech and language skills of adults with Down syndrome. In J.F. Miller, M. Leddy and L.A. Leavitt (eds), *Improving the Communication of People with Down Syndrome*. Baltimore: Paul H. Brookes, pp. 205–213.

Lenneberg, E. (1967) *Biological Foundations of Language*. New York: Wiley.

Rondal, J.A. (2003) Appendix 1: Major acquisitions in morphosyntactic development. In J.A. Rondal and S. Buckley (eds), *Speech and Language Intervention in Down Syndrome*. London: Whurr.

Rondal, J.A. and Buckley, S. (eds) (2003) *Speech and Language Intervention in Down Syndrome*. London: Whurr.

Sackett, D.L., Richardson, W.S., Rosenberg, W.M.C. and Haynes, R.B. (1997) *Evidence-based Medicine: How to Practice and Teach EBM*. London: Churchill Livingstone.

30

Bridging the research–clinical divide through postgraduate research training

Georgia D. Bertou

Speech and Language Therapist, Athens, Greece

As a paediatric speech and language therapist (SLT), there are many challenges to working in an evidence-based way. This chapter describes my journey from working clinically in the UK, to practising and researching in Greece. I will describe my choice to undertake a postgraduate degree (Master of Science; MSc) in order to develop the necessary skills to use research in my practice more effectively and to develop further as a clinician.

After graduating as an SLT, I spent one year practising in the UK. Along the way, I found that I had many questions about language acquisition, the meaning of words, the organization of the lexicon and the importance of these factors to the development of overall language skills and later literacy skills. My interest in this particular area was strengthened while I was working for the National Health Service in community clinics, where, based on my readings of associated research and on my clinical practice, I could see the important role of lexical knowledge/ vocabulary skills on children's language and literacy skills. I wanted to undertake research that would combine both practical and theoretical issues so that it would be useful to therapists and researchers. An important factor for me was that I planned to eventually practise in Greece, where I was born. Therefore, I felt that my research should be something that was relevant to the Greek population.

When exploring the options for postgraduate study, I found that there were several possible pathways. Some Masters courses offered the opportunity to specialize/focus on a single area of clinical practice academically. However, I felt that I had burning questions that I wanted to answer myself using a process of research. I also wanted to be actively involved in research following my degree, and to be able to follow an academic or research career in the future.

Vocabulary development in Greek children

Vocabulary development is one of the areas of speech and language therapy that has not been sufficiently investigated in Greece. The vast majority of research has focused on the description of linguistic properties of Greek language such as morphology rather than language acquisition. Several studies have focused on syntactic and grammatical development (Katis, 1984, cited in Maridaki-Kassotaki *et al.*, 2003; Varlokosta, 1996; Tsimpli, 2001). However, language acquisition has not been targeted by researchers with the same enthusiasm, resulting in few studies on this area (Manolitsis, 2000). Additionally, most published studies on vocabulary acquisition have been limited to English language speakers, thus any conclusions on early lexical acquisition in Greek children would be premature due to the lack of systematic empirical studies on large enough corpora. In contrast there has been a great amount of research on the development, assessment and therapy of phonological difficulties and the role of phonological processes on the development of reading, writing and generally school performance (Aidinis and Nunes, 2001; Kotoulas, 2003; Yianetopoulou, 2003). In the field of child speech and language disorders, there are at least two published tests assessing phonological (Levadi, Kirpotin *et al.*, 1995) and meta-phonological development (Yianetopoulou and Kirpotin, 2007) that have been statistically standardized on the Greek population; but none on language skills such as reception of grammar, expressive syntax or receptive vocabulary. These areas are covered briefly by subsections of tests used mainly by educational psychologists for the detection of learning difficulties (Paraskevopoulos *et al.*, 1999), as well as screening tools which are very useful to detect difficulties on those areas and to assess school readiness, but not to set therapy targets and to monitor therapy effectiveness (Panhellenic Association of Logopedists, 2005).

I believe that psychometric tests can be a valuable tool for therapists and researchers. As a clinical therapist I found the use of standardized assessments very helpful in the assessment of children's skills, in the assessment of therapy efficacy and in monitoring children's progress in order to set new goals. A lack of standardized formal assessments causes considerable challenges in the identification of such difficulties. I wanted to address this problem by developing a reliable and valid vocabulary assessment for Greek school age children.

My research project was an experimental study to measure both receptive and expressive vocabulary of Greek children aged six to eight years. The results provide preliminary data to facilitate the future development of a standardized, reliable test for Greek vocabulary (Bertou, 2005). I presented the findings of my project at the 'Realising the Vision' conference of the Royal College of Speech and Language Therapists in Belfast in May 2006 (Bertou, 2006). I received useful comments, advice and encouragement to continue the development of the vocabulary test from other therapists and researchers.

My current practice

I am currently working as a SLT in Athens in four different paediatric settings. I work as part of a multidisciplinary team at a private school for children with autism and profound and multiple learning disabilities (PMLD). I also work at a private clinic with children with a variety of speech and language difficulties and I provide home visits. Additionally I work at a developmental assessment unit, at the P. & A. Kyriakou Children's Hospital in Athens. Working in the private sector has given me the opportunity to work in different settings and explore areas of clinical interest.

In 2006 I started working at the Developmental Assessment Unit of Athens University as a part-time research assistant. This Unit operates both as a child development assessment unit and as a research centre. It offers the opportunity to researchers of different educational and professional backgrounds to collaborate and study aspects of child development. Through this role, I have had the opportunity to further develop my research skills whilst working with other researchers on several projects that will be of considerable benefit to the SLT profession, and to associated disciplines, in Greece. The first was exploring cognitive and behavioural abilities of children with human immunodeficiency virus (HIV) infection. Although the sample was small, the findings of this study supported the idea that HIV infection places children at increased risk for poor cognitive and behavioural outcomes only if they experience a severe illness of advancing disease stage or a coexisting disease. This study was presented at the 25th International Congress of Pediatrics in Athens in August 2007. This study was placed in the two hundred best abstracts by the Congress scientific committee and was published online in the American Journal *Pediatrics* in the Supplement of January 2008 (Bertou *et al.*, 2008). Ongoing research with a larger group of children, is investigating factors that influence the behaviour and self-esteem of children with HIV infection.

I have also participated in the development of the 'A TEST' which is a screening tool for children's school readiness in Greece (Thomaidis and Mantoudis, 2006). This test is now being used widely in Greece by pediatricians, educational psychologists, SLTs and occupational therapists. The long-term aim of the multidisciplinary team involved in this study is for the 'A TEST' to gain the recognition of the Greek government and to be administered in all state schools, free of charge as a standard procedure. This will help enormously in the early identification of possible literacy and behaviour difficulties.

Reflections on the MSc as a pathway to being a clinician–researcher

Before I joined the MSc programme I thought that the most important thing that I would gain from this experience would be to address my clinical question around vocabulary development in Greek children through the research project. However, when I completed the course and returned to clinical practice I realized that I was mistaken. What I have learned in terms of critically analysing, 'filtering' and applying research to practice has been the most important learning to me as a clinician. These skills are what make it feasible for me to be 'evidence-based' in my own practice.

As far as research is concerned, I have been exposed to critical issues of qualitative and quantitative research in speech and language therapy and in methods of implementing research in professional practice. I have been introduced to a wide range of methodologies and analysis techniques in order to choose the ones that are suitable for a research project. I have developed several practical skills needed to design and conduct a research project, such as deciding on the appropriate study design, hypothesis setting, ethical research practice, developing and administering a methodology, collecting data and compiling a database, reporting, analysing and interpreting data, citing and formatting references. These have been vital in the research that I have subsequently been involved in.

Today, I consider myself firstly a clinician and then a junior researcher. The research that I undertake will always be oriented toward clinical practice. I feel proud of the fact that my MSc project is one of the first steps towards the development of a standardized reliable and valid assessment of vocabulary in Greek, and that the data that I collected can be useful in the Greek research field, as a useful starting point for further research.

I feel that my experience of the student research for my MSc has helped me to gain new skills as well as confidence to continue looking for opportunities to be research-active whilst working as a clinician. My current experiences of working as part of a multidisciplinary research team have highlighted the value that can be added by combining a range of different perspectives to address a shared clinical question. I am also continuing to learn from working alongside more experienced researchers.

I continue to feel strongly that all our patients deserve to be offered assessment, treatment and therapy techniques that have been proven to be effective. I also feel that we all have a duty as clinicians to add to the body of evidence that underpins our practice for the ultimate benefit of our profession and our patients. Barriers and difficulties in adopting a culture of evidence-based practice (EBP) within the SLT profession are inevitable, irrespective of the therapist's cultural/educational background. In the case of a limited evidence base, it is important not to use the lack of research as an excuse for not trying to stay as close as possible to engaging in EBP. On the contrary, I think that it can be seen as inspiration and as a challenge to be faced: it can be hard work but it is certainly rewarding.

Acknowledgements

I would like to thank Dr Hazel Roddam and Dr Jemma Skeat, editors of this book, as well as Dr Thomaidis, Assistant Professor at the Developmental Assessment Unit of Athens University at P. & A. Kyriakou Children's Hospital, plus my MSc research project supervisor at the University of Sheffield, Dr Marcin Szczerbinski.

References

Aidinis, A. and Nunes, T. (2001) The role of different levels of phonological awareness in the development of reading and spelling in Greek. *Reading and Writing: An Interdisciplinary Journal*, **14**, 145–177.

Bertou, G. (2005) The development of a receptive and expressive vocabulary test for 6–8-year-old Greek children. Unpublished Masters Thesis, University of Sheffield, UK.

Bertou, G. (2006) The development of a receptive and expressive vocabulary test for 6–8 year old Greek children. Paper presented at the RCSLT Conference, Ulster, May 2006.

Bertou, G., Thomaidis, L., Spoulou, V. and Theodoridou, M. (2008) Cognitive and behavioural abilities of children with HIV infection in Greece. *Pediatrics*, **121** (Suppl 2), S100.

Kotoulas, B. (2003) Phonemic awareness and reading difficulties. *Language*, **56**, 29–50.

Levadi, E., Kirpotin, L., Kardamitsi, E. and Kabouroglou, M. (1995) *Test of Phonetic and Phonological Development*. Athens: Panhellenic Association of Logopedists.

Manolitsis, G. (2000) *Assessment of Meta-linguistic Abilities of Children between 5–6 Years of Age*. Athens: Grigoris Publications.

Maridaki-Kassotaki, K., Lewis, C. and Freeman, N.H. (2003) Lexical choice can lead to problems; What false-belief tests tell us about Greek alternative verbs of agency. *Journal of Child Language*, 30, 145–164.

Panhellenic Association of Logopedists (2005) *Anomilo 4 Test for the Detection of Speech and Language Difficulties of Children of Four Years of Age*. Athens: Ellinika Grammata.

Paraskevopoulos, I., Kalazi-Azizi, A. and Gianitsas, N. (1999) *Athina Test for the Diagnosis of Learning Difficulties*. Athens: Ellinika Grammata.

Thomaidis, L. and Mantoudis, S. (2006) *A'Test: Screening Test of School Readiness*. Athens: Anaptiski.

Tsimpli, I.M. (2001) Interpretability and language development: A study of verbal and nominal features in greek normally developing and SLI children. *Brain and Language*, 77 (3), 432–448.

Varlokosta, S. (1996) Optional infinitives in child language. *Studies in Greek Linguistics*, 18, 297–308.

Yianetopoulou, A. (2003) From speaking to writing: Research on the development of phonological awareness in Greek language. In M. Glikas and G. Kalomiris (eds), *Communication and Speech Disorders*. Athens: Ellinika Grammata, pp. 144–169.

Yianetopoulou, A. and Kirpotin, L. (2007) *Metaphon Test: A Standardised Tool of Metaphonological Development and Reading Readiness*. Athens: Grigoris Publications.

31

Many roads lead to EBP (commentary on Section Five)

Jemma Skeat and Hazel Roddam

When planning this book, we felt that it was important to include examples of clinician's individual experiences in implementing evidence in practice, showcasing the diversity of how this happens in real life. The 'textbook' approach to evidence-based practice (EBP) is to identify a clinical problem, evaluate the evidence, apply the evidence, and evaluate the changes. The clinical examples in this section illustrate that, in reality, each of these steps happens in diverse ways. Speech and language therapists (SLTs) are using EBP as a problem-solving tool, and also as a proactive approach to guide decision-making in practice. The way that they approach the literature varies, and these examples illustrate diverse strategies to facilitate the often time-consuming task of identifying and evaluating the relevant evidence. The amount and level of evidence that they found was also variable, which is the reality for our profession. Nevertheless, in these examples clinicians were able to use what existed, along with their clinical judgement and patient preferences, in order to make decisions about practice – illustrating what Roddam (2004) argued is 'evidence-informed' practice. This is what EBP is all about, and these examples illustrate that even though we all follow the same basic map, the roads to EBP are many and varied.

Defining a clinical question

Guyatt and Meade (2008) suggest that clinical questions are developed on the basis of a 'clinical dilemma'; that is, a clinical situation where the best way to proceed is unclear. Our chapters illustrate two different types of clinical dilemmas that may prompt a clinical question.

Dilemma 1: Things are not working

When therapy appears to be ineffective or potentially impacts negatively on other areas such as patient quality of life, clinicians face a 'clinical dilemma'. An example of this is Chapter 26 where Beth and Linda noted that a group of patients were not responding to traditional voice therapy offered in their service. Their challenge was to consider alternative approaches and to look at the evidence that existed to support those options. Amanda and Leora (Chapter 27) similarly faced a dilemma in the use of thickened fluids with residents in a nursing home, which was impacting negatively on residents' quality of life.

Dilemma 2: Facing unfamiliar territory

Even very experienced clinicians may be faced with a clinical dilemma in the shape of a client (or group of clients) with an unfamiliar problem, where the next steps for assessment/diagnosis, prognosis, and therapy are not clear. For Shalini (Chapter 20), the assessment and therapy provision for older children with limited language development, in a context of limited therapy resources, presented 'unfamiliar territory'.

Other approaches

On the other hand, waiting for a 'clinical dilemma' to rear its head is not the only way that clinical questions are prompted, as our authors demonstrate. External events – such as the publication of new guidelines (Chapter 25) or the development of a new service (Chapter 22) – may prompt the need for SLTs to review the evidence and implement changes. Some questions are also prompted by reflecting on current practices, perhaps even those that are very familiar and comfortable, proactively examining practice in order to justify current approaches or identify best practice alternatives. Two examples of taking a second look at current practices for familiar problems are Chapter 21, where Angela, Catherine and Parimala reviewed the evidence around the participation of children using AAC, and Chapter 24, where Anneli re-examined how best to facilitate treatment carry-over from the clinic to the home and school for children with autism.

Identifying and appraising the evidence

Having a clinical question in mind, all of the contributing authors in this section accessed the evidence, but not all underwent a 'traditional' literature review process. For example, in Chapter 29, Ruth discussed the use of pre-appraised literature sources by students on clinical placements. These resources, such as book chapters, guidelines, and critically appraised papers can provide a concise, clear summary of the best evidence, sometimes geared towards the clinical bottom line (Haynes, 2001), which can be an enormous help to a busy clinician or student with limited appraisal skills (Straus and McAlister, 2000). However, not all of the sources available to clinicians present rigourous evidence. Some are not designed to do this, and McKibbon *et al.* (2008) highlight that clinicians need to consider whether their chosen resource provides evidence, as compared to clinical opinion and conjecture. For example, does the resource cite the evidence used to form its assertions/conclusions, and is the strength of that evidence discussed?

For clinicians undertaking a wider review themselves, several strategies used in these chapters are worth highlighting. Angela, Catherine and Parimala (Chapter 21) shared the task of evaluating the literature among senior staff (including a clinician–researcher) and clinical SLTs. Shared appraisal may provide an opportunity for clinical staff with less experience or knowledge about research evidence appraisal to be exposed to the process with scaffolding and support from more experienced colleagues (Straus and McAlister, 2000). In this case, the department started with a question that was agreed to be important to their clinical practice, and which would have a real life impact – rather than a hypothetical case or scenario. They suggested that having clinicians involved in the process was crucial to their success in implementing the changes, because there was ownership of the process and the conclusions that they made. Sharing appraisal of the literature also reduces the individual load required to pursue evidence-based answers to clinical questions.

The use of existing resources is important. Angela, Catherine and Parimala made use of the clinician–researcher post to undertake the initial literature search for the department. As literature searching may be daunting, making use of people who already have well-developed skills to undertake this part of the EBP process may be a good starting point. An alternative may be to partner with researchers in other institutes, which is what a Swedish SLT decided to do when she contacted Christina (Chapter 28). Christina, who has a university post, undertook the literature review and provided guidance for the clinician in implementing the evidence, and in adding to the evidence-base through a research project. Daniel and Gracie (Chapter 25) made use of on-site support for literature searching through their hospital library. Many other SLTs may feel that they have enhanced their skills in research appraisal by undertaking further formal education which includes a research focus, as Georgia did in Chapter 30. Georgia reflects that this approach has provided a strong basis for her use of evidence in practice today:

> What I have learned in terms of critically analysing, 'filtering' and applying research to practice has been the most important learning to me as a clinician. These skills are what make it feasible for me to be 'evidence-based' in my own practice (p. 203).

Georgia's experience is her own, and we don't suggest that this route is for everyone. Nevertheless, for those who specifically wish to develop strong research and EBP skills, or postgraduate education programmes may be an option worth considering.

Finally, Patricia's discussion of EBP in the case of Alex, a young boy with a stutter growing up in a bilingual home (Chapter 23), demonstrates that EBP is not just about searching the research literature. Patricia used the research evidence alongside other important tools for clinical decision-making: her case history and clinical observations about Alex and his parents, and her discussions with Alex and his parents. The importance of taking into account the needs, expectations and preferences of clients and families has always been part of EBP (Sackett et al., 1996), and the related patient/client/family-centred practice movement has also emphasized the value of these perspectives (Rosenbaum et al., 1998).

Implementing the evidence

When the evidence indicates a need to change current practice, clinicians face the challenge of actually implementing these changes. Implementing the evidence can be particularly complicated when large changes are needed and/or when multiple stakeholders are involved or affected. Angela, Catherine and Parimala (Chapter 21) needed to address both of these issues. The service changes that they implemented challenged the assumptions of stakeholders about the best way to provide services for children using AAC in schools. Nevertheless, with the evidence to support them, they were able to negotiate these changes with a wide range of stakeholders – including SLTs, therapy managers, other professional staff in their organization, government agencies, university faculties, teachers, clients and families.

The level of change and the number of stakeholders involved may not be the only issues that impact on implementation. Sometimes existing resources simply do not support the changes required. For Daniel and Gracie (Chapter 25), therapist time to implement communication therapy was challenged by competing priorities in the acute setting. Their practical, flexible approach was to provide activities to be undertaken independently by clients (with the support of families) where possible, and to make use of an allied health assistant. Although unable to realign practice fully with the recommended two hours per week suggested in the literature, Daniel and Gracie managed to make changes so that practice better reflected the research evidence in their service.

Evaluating changes

Evaluating change is an essential part of EBP. Without this, the 'cycle' is not complete – we don't know if we have accomplished what we set out to when we developed the clinical question in the first place. Examples in these chapters ranged from informal reflection on changes to clinical practice and the potential positive and negative outcomes of these, to more formal evaluations where data were purposefully collected and examined, in some cases as small research projects. There are just a few points that we would like to highlight from these examples.

First, evaluation should take into account multiple perspectives. Clinicians, clients, parents, and other stakeholders may all have different (positive or negative) views about the changes that have been made. In some situations, these perspectives may be the only way of understanding the real impact of changes. For example, getting teacher and parent views is key to understanding how a new therapy approach is supporting children at home and in the classroom (see Anneli's Chapter 24).

Shalini (Chapter 20) illustrates another important point – that evaluation needs to examine whether the way that evidence has been applied meets local cultural and social needs, and is sustainable and practical with respect to resources. These reflections may suggest the need to rethink strategies for applying the evidence, or the need to go back to look for other evidence-based approaches that do fit with the local situation.

Finally, some of our authors reflected that their evaluation could have benefited from early planning. For example, Daniel and Gracie (Chapter 25) stated that they felt that data about the number of communication sessions that clients received and client satisfaction with therapy should have been collected, in order to demonstrate that communication therapy was feasible and valuable. It can be difficult to try and identify potential process and outcome measures from the start; however without this forward thinking there is nothing to demonstrate the hard work that you have done and the progress that has been made. Considering the aims and likely outcomes of the changes that you want to implement is fundamental to planning a good evaluation strategy. Further discussion around evaluation can be found in Section Six of this book.

Summary

The chapters in this section illustrate that local resources, pressures, opportunities and stakeholders, as well as the evidence that is available, all influence how the processes of EBP are applied. EBP is not a 'formula' that follows the same path every time. There are many roads to EBP, although it is important to keep the destination in mind: the use of research evidence, patient preferences and clinical knowledge to guide decision making in practice (Sackett *et al.*, 1996). We hope that these diverse examples will provide encouragement for you to consider different ways that you can undertake EBP in your service.

References

Guyatt, G. and Meade, M. (2008) How to use the medical literature- and this book- to improve your patient care. In G. Guyatt (ed.), *User's Guides to the Medical Literature: Essentials for Evidence-Based Clinical Practice*. New York: McGraw-Hill Professional.

Haynes, R.B. (2001) Of studies, syntheses, synopses and systems: the 4S evolution of services for finding current best evidence. *ACP Journal Club*, **134** (2), A11–A13.

McKibbon, A., Wyer, P., Jaeschke, R. and Hunt, D. (2008) Finding the evidence. In G. Guyatt (ed.), *User's Guides to the Medical Literature: Essentials for Evidence-Based Clinical Practice*. New York: McGraw-Hill Professional, pp. 32–76.

Roddam, H. (2004) The efficacy of augmentative and alternative communication: Towards evidence-based practice (Editorial). *Communication Matters*, **18** (2), 23–24.

Rosenbaum, P., King, S., Law, M., King, G. and Evans, J. (1998) Family-centred service: A conceptual framework and research review. *Physical and Occupational Therapy in Pediatrics*, **18** (1), 1–20.

Sackett, D.L., Rosenberg, W.M.C., Gray, J.A.M., Haynes, R.B. and Richardson, W.S. (1996) Evidence based medicine: What it is and what it isn't. *British Medical Journal*, **312** (7023), 71–72.

Straus, S.E. and McAlister, F.A. (2000) Evidence-based medicine: A commentary on common criticisms. *Canadian Medical Association Journal*, **163** (7), 837–841.

Section Six

Future directions for EBP in speech and language therapy

32

Wider consultation on embedding EBP in SLT practice

Hazel Roddam and Jemma Skeat

The examples provided in this book are only some of potentially hundreds of approaches that speech and language therapists (SLTs) are taking to embed evidence based practice (EBP) in their own local settings. One of the key aims of this book is to encourage sharing of approaches to EBP across clinicians. One of the ways in which we extended this beyond those who were invited contributors to the book was to hold a workshop during the research symposium at the Royal College of Speech and Language Therapists International Scientific Conference in London, 2009. The workshop asked participants to share the ways that they embed EBP. The themes arising from this workshop were varied – and many complemented those that have already been developed by the authors in this book. This chapter briefly discusses some of these themes, particularly those which we hope may suggest some additional ideas or considerations for embedding EBP. It particularly includes discussion about the role of the professional bodies in supporting EBP. We believe that these bodies have a key role to play in moving the profession forward, and were keen to understand how participants perceived this role. Before we report the results of the workshop, we will give some background as to the process that we undertook.

Workshop process

The workshop began with a short introduction to EBP, with brief illustrations of some of the themes that have come out of the contributed chapters. Participants then had the opportunity to individually reflect and record their own responses to three prompts.

- Things I do to embed EBP
- Things my service does to embed EBP
- Comments on the role of the professional bodies to support embedding EBP.

After a few moments, we asked participants to contribute ideas from their own personal list and these ideas were recorded for the group under those three headings. Participants were able to clarify ideas or initiatives volunteered by other people, but the principal aim was to generate substantive lists of examples, rather than to engage in immediate discussion of each item in turn. The process used in the workshop for individually recording and then sharing ideas was based on the Nominal Group Technique (Bartunek and Murnighan, 1984; Potter *et al.*, 2004). Ideally, this process would have included sharing until the group had exhausted all of the ideas on their individual lists. In anticipation that there would be insufficient time to achieve this, we invited participants to submit their individual lists to us at the end of the session so that we could capture a record of the remaining items. In order to get an idea about the diversity of the fields and places of practice represented in the group, participants were also asked to indicate these.

Approximately 80 delegates attended this workshop. A total of 32 participants submitted their individual lists at the end of the meeting. Participants reflected a wide range of clinical backgrounds, representing adult and paediatric community services, mental health, schools services and hospitals, and working in diverse areas including early language, voice, dysphagia, learning disabilities, acquired brain injury, craniofacial conditions and hearing impairment. All participants who provided their details were from the UK (representing England, Northern Ireland and Wales) and the Republic of Ireland. The lists provided by each participant, as well as the examples provided by the larger group during the workshop, were coded into themes for each of the prompts above.

Embedding EBP: what clinicians and services are doing

The output from the first two question prompts of the workshop was synthesized into themes, as shown in Box 32.1.

We cannot discuss in detail all of the themes shown in Box 32.1, many of which have been described or touched upon in previous chapters from our contributors. However, we wanted to take this opportunity to reflect on some of the key issues that arose, particularly those that gave new perspectives.

Learning and practising EBP skills

The importance of knowledge and skills in EBP is a key theme throughout this book. The participants in this workshop echoed this theme, suggesting that training and development opportunities are vital for them to approach EBP with confidence and with the necessary skills and abilities. Access to learning opportunities was an important way that services support EBP. Colleagues are clearly an important resource for EBP, both as sources of information and as sounding boards to consider clinical problems and the evidence. Several chapters in this book have highlighted the importance of peer communication and support in relation to EBP in big and small ways. The workshop participants confirmed that they recognized the importance of peer support. Strategies used by workshop participants to gain confidence through colleagues included:

- seeking specialist advice for an identified issue
- case discussion with colleagues to support routine clinical decision-making about patient care

Box 32.1   Themes arising from the workshop illustrating 'Things I do to embed EBP' and 'Things my service does to embed EBP'

Things I do to embed EBP

Seeking training and development
- *Attending conference/special interest groups (SIGs)/training/journal clubs*
- *Arranged EBP SIG session – Dysphagia in adults with learning difficulties (ALD)*
- *Attend SIGs and conferences*

Learning and sharing with colleagues
- *Shadowing colleagues/specialists– tertiary centres*
- *Pass on information/findings and discuss with others in my consultancy role*
- *Discuss cases/groups in supervision to find out what others know*
- *Appraising research jointly with peers/colleagues from other professions*

Being research active and embedding findings into practice
- *Currently studying for an MPhil*
- *Started a research project in dysphagia prevalence in a learning difficulties (LD) population*

Translating primary research into recommendations for clinical practice
- *Agree care packages/pathways for my area of clinical practice based on published research/agreed management, i.e. from SIGs, etc.*
- *Review guidelines (and update)*
- *Ensure that service design and implementation takes into account the evidence base*

Involving clients in practice
- *Seek client view and table developments to a parent forum*
- *Obtain parental and professional feedback on outcomes*

Utilizing existing resources
- *Use library service*
- *Use RCSLT clinical guidelines*
- *Refer to evidence-based care pathways*

Taking time to reflect
- *Schedule time in working week to reflect on my own practice*
- *Specifically record how effective I am finding using cervical auscultation as a tool with young children*
- *Read journal articles – any new ideas?*
- *Audit against evidenced standards – e.g. accessible information*

Things my service does to embed EBP

Facilitating learning and sharing with colleagues
- *Provides case discussion mornings to discuss examples of good practice*

- *Key person who has a role in pulling out relevant articles to read*
- *Multidisciplinary clinical review and projects with reflective practice*

Providing support for training and development
- *Support requests for external training to keep up to date with EBP in particular clinical fields*
- *All staff have ½ session per month to do continuing professional development (CPD)*
- *Structure and framework to support new graduate clinicians in EBP*

Providing encouragement and support for research and evaluation
- *Encourage clinicians to apply for research secondment programmes*
- *Links with all London universities*
- *Biannual 'celebrating success' conference takes place to celebrate projects/ research. Multidisciplinary audience invited, including parents*

Providing resources to support EBP within practice
- *Access to library resources/databases on computer*
- *Collecting articles into a service database of relevant topics*
- *Write standard operating procedures using EBP*

Supporting dissemination of research and evaluation
- *Makes time for writing of papers/presentations*
- *Holds study days for Early Years practitioners (SLTs, teachers and assistants) – venue for disseminating research findings and discussing EBP*

- shared appraisal of research literature and discussion/ debate about research findings and their application to practice.

Participants also suggested value in seeking this support not just from SLTs, but from colleagues in other disciplines. They were clear that there are many things that services are doing to facilitate this peer support, including team meetings, journal clubs, multidisciplinary case discussion, and providing time to shadow colleagues.

Research activity

As discussed earlier, it is not the intended message of this book to encourage SLTs to embark on a research career in order to embed EBP. Nevertheless, several contributors have highlighted the importance of research activity in building skills and knowledge, and in adding to the evidence base. A number of workshop participants also reported that they had either enrolled or had completed higher degrees, or that they were currently research active themselves. It is natural that as clinicians become more confident in appraising research evidence and applying it in their own routine practice, that they may become more motivated to evaluate the success of their own clinical interventions in a structured, scientific way. Thus, EBP becomes cyclical, as clinicians both use and contribute to the literature in their field. By undertaking well-designed and well-conducted small-scale studies, experienced clinicians could make highly valuable contributions to the collective professional evidence base. Contact and collaboration with local universities and contacts with SLTs who have greater experience in research may be useful to support this process, and this was certainly suggested by workshop participants. We would like to emphasize the point, however, that you do not have to register for a research degree to become research-active: you simply have to begin undertaking systematic evaluations of your own clinical practice, preferably with advice from a colleague who already has relevant research experience.

Developing or using evidence-based resources for clinical practice

A number of the workshop participants reported that their services are actively engaged in writing local protocols for national clinical guidelines, or in designing evidence-based patient pathways. Others reported that their teams collate resource files of research evidence so that it is easily accessible to all staff, or aim to maximize the use of existing resources, such as the published clinical guideline sets developed by professional bodies such as RCSLT. These initiatives would all appear to be effective strategies for supporting the implementation of research evidence into local clinical practice; as well as promoting the standardization of the local service delivery.

Maximizing the use of existing resources to support EBP

This was a valuable theme which was raised and reinforced by workshop participants. Practical examples were cited of resources that SLTs had found to be valuable, both in terms of being time efficient, plus affirming that they were implementing good clinical practice. Local examples of assistance from medical librarians were given, including instances where this is provided as a ward-round service. Other examples of more widely available sources of evidence-based clinical guidelines may serve as a valuable reminder as demonstrated by several of our contributors, that we should always look first for these pre-appraised sources of evidence, before we undertake to start hunting for primary studies.

Involving clients

We were delighted to note that participants listed examples of ways in which they actively engage with their service users as an integral element of the approach to EBP. Individuals reported talking with their own clients about their perceptions of the therapy outcomes. A number of the workshop participants additionally reported service-wide initiatives either to consult with service users, or to involve them in showcase events to celebrate good practice in collaborative working. It is naturally important that such events are planned and conducted in a considered and sensitive way.

Taking time to reflect

In the course of the workshop the theme of reflective practice was raised more explicitly than has been discussed in our previous chapters. Many of the participants referred to reflective practice, in addition to a number of related practical strategies. We acknowledge that this topic merits more in-depth consideration, particularly to try to understand what reflective practice means to SLTs, and how it can directly support EBP. The following chapter picks up this theme and also links it to other ways in which we can review our clinical practice.

Comments on the role of professional bodies

The workshop provided us with an opportunity to invite comments on the role of professional bodies, such as the Royal College of Speech and Language Therapists, Speech Pathology Australia, the American Speech–Language–Hearing Association (ASHA), and others around the world, in supporting individuals and services to become more evidence based. This is not a theme that has been discussed in any detail by authors in this book; nevertheless, the influence of the professional bodies can be seen to underpin some of the initiatives and approaches described in this book, including the following examples.

*   The redevelopment of the speech and language therapy curriculum developed at Hanze University (Chapter 4) was a response to the Dutch Association of Logopedics and Phoniatrics (NVLF) updating their profile for SLTs, which led to new competency standards that emphasized EBP;
*   Siân and Tracey (Chapter 12) highlight the role of the RCSLT in promoting EBP in the UK through *Communicating Quality* (RCSLT, 2006) and in published clinical guidelines (RCSLT, 2005) which collate for SLTs the current evidence base for interventions;
*   Several authors, including Angie (Chapter 17) have utilized the guidelines, position papers and other publications from professional associations when considering the evidence base and/or seeking previous clinical recommendations in a particular area.

The themes arising from the workshop highlight some of these existing initiatives and suggest still others. These themes, with some illustrative examples of each, are provided in Box 32.2. It is worth considering whether these themes reflect what is currently happening in the professional bodies, or whether they are challenges for the professional bodies to meet into the future. We suspect that there is a wide variance in what professional bodies are doing around the world, and that while some of these roles may have been largely acknowledged and addressed, others may pose fresh challenges.

Setting the strategic agenda and facilitating the development of evidence

The participants noted that the professional bodies have a role that sits across clinical areas, specialties and settings, and with links to both policy and practice. The potential therefore, is for professional bodies to take a strategic view of EBP: identifying the 'missing pieces' of evidence that would move the profession forward. This may include advocating for the use of methodologies that will support the use of evidence in practice (for example, systematic reviews), and tying this together with current policy directions. Related to this was a call for increased practical

> **Box 32.2   Themes arising from the workshop illustrating participant's comments on the role of professional bodies in supporting EBP**
>
> Comments on the role of the professional bodies to support embedding EBP
>
> Setting a strategic agenda to promote and support EBP
> - *Leading on influencing research finding and directions*
> - *Set up focus groups involving users, service providers and academics to decide what the key questions to be answered are*
> - *Use the UK CRC research classification system (or similar) to plan research priorities for the profession*
>
> Supporting the development of the evidence base
> - *Building up a knowledge base to share*
> - *Guidance on attracting funding*
> - *Negotiate with research funding bodies to raise the profile of (systematic) reviews*
>
> Sharing information about new evidence
> - *Information on what has been published and where for various clinical areas- perhaps through clinical networks?*
> - *Reviews/updates in RCSLT Bulletin i.e. 'best practice'*
> - *Managers network to publicize EBP and share good models of incorporating EBP.*
>
> Providing guidance and training for conducting EBP
> - *Accredited training.*
> - *Developing competency levels.*
> - *Guidelines on how to do EBP, e.g. easy guide to EBP*
> - *Research advisor in RCSLT*

support for the development of the evidence base. Participants suggested that the professional bodies could do this through providing funding themselves, advocating for government or other funding sources to focus on issues relevant to SLTs, or simply by more clearly signposting existing funding sources.

Communicating the message: disseminating new evidence, training and resources

A number of examples raised in the workshop indicated ways in which the professional bodies could more actively communicate the evidence with members (including through dissemination and through training), and also encourage communication across the wider membership. There was a wealth of proposals around maximizing opportunities for the active dissemination of new research information. Some of the suggestions included utilizing existing channels, including Special Interest Groups and networks of Specialist Clinical Advisors. Professional magazines and other widely-read bulletins were advocated for hosting regular reviews of evidence for best practice, as well as for alerts to key research publications in peer-reviewed journals. It was also proposed that the potential for electronic media could be maximized. On-line discussion forums dedicated to research reviews were particularly advocated, and it was suggested that professional association websites could provide a forum for researchers to highlight the clinical implications and applications of their work.

Training needs have already been discussed more generally throughout the book. However, it is worth highlighting that participants saw a specific role for the professional bodies in providing training opportunities. The extent to which professional bodies are able to provide training opportunities may vary across countries, but provision of CPD events or short courses is not the only way to meet the needs within the profession and to skill them up in EBP. Providing a central point of access to or recommendations around short courses, CPD opportunities and EBP resources, which may include online tutorials and 'beginner guides' to EBP is a useful starting point. These resources and training opportunities do not have to be developed or necessarily run by the professional bodies, nor do they have to be SLT specific in order to be useful.

Many professional associations have started the process of communicating the message through key documents summarizing the evidence and providing clinical guidelines for practice, plus through the provision of online resources or links to external resources. For example, ASHA have a number of initiatives providing online resources, guidance and summaries of evidence for members, as well as some web-based tutorials on EBP concepts and skills. The Italian Federation of Speech and Language Therapists (FLI) has recently launched a collaborative initiative with the Officina Napoli Cochrane (ONC), with the aim of delivering multi-disciplinary training in EBP. The initiative to date incorporates SLTs, physiotherapists, nurses and physicians. With the emphasis on promoting integrated professional working practices, they aim to focus on the relevant professional research literature to develop evidence-based guidelines for clinical practice.

Some professional associations have endorsement or accreditation processes for CPD courses, by way of quality assurance. Participants suggested that part of this accreditation of training should be to ensure that training includes explicit links to the relevant evidence base, as well as emphasizing the relevant multidisciplinary evidence bases, in recognition that SLTs work across professional boundaries and very often in multidisciplinary teams.

Summary

The initiatives, approaches and examples suggested by our workshop participants and summarized here present some excellent additional suggestions for embedding EBP in SLT practice. One of the aims of this book was to provide a forum for sharing of individual and service initiatives, and it has been exciting to see how the themes that are discussed by our contributors have been mirrored in the workshop. What we have found, both through our contributors and through the workshop, is that SLTs are embedding EBP in creative, strategic ways that make use of their local services and settings and we hope that these provide some ideas to start or to enhance the ways that other SLTs can also embed EBP.

There are many excellent initiatives underway world-wide across the respective professional associations. However, these are not always optimally highlighted. We feel it is essential for the professional bodies to have the opportunity to consider the perspectives of their members regarding their role in EBP; some of these suggestions may be already well underway, others may be challenges that need to be met in the future.

Most of the workshop participants were from the UK. Nevertheless, the clinicians who attended reflected a wide range of clinical backgrounds and levels of experience in relation to clinical practice, EBP and research activity. We are currently exploring opportunities for consultation with SLTs internationally.

Acknowledgements

We would like to thank and acknowledge all of the participants in the RCSLT workshop in March 2009, including the following clinicians who provided their names: Daphne Banat, Anna Collins, Teresa Dilley, Annabel Edwards, Lisa Everton, Alison Fuller, Deb Gibbard, Juliet Goldbart, Alison Hudson, Cathy Johnston, Dierdre Kenny, Clare Keohane, Sarah Mason, Valerie Pereiv, Emma Philp, Louisa Reeves, Carol Sacchett, Chris Salis, C Shipster, Bryony Simpson, Clare Smith, Nina Soloff, Kristianne Stewart, Juan Titteringten, Sarah Todder, Kim Turner, Cath Valentine.

References

Bartunek, J.M. and Murnighan, J.K. (1984) The nominal group technique: Expanding the basic procedure and underlying assumptions. *Group and Organization Studies*, **9**, 417–432.

Potter, M., Gordon, S. and Hamer, P. (2004) The nominal group technique: A useful consensus methodology in physiotherapy research. *New Zealand Journal of Physiotherapy*, **32** (3), 126–130.

Royal College of Speech and Language Therapists (2005) *Clinical Guidelines*. Oxon: Speechmark.

Royal College of Speech and Language Therapists (2006) *Communicating quality* (3rd edn). London: RCSLT.

33

The role of reflective practice in supporting EBP

Jemma Skeat and Hazel Roddam

We would like to use this chapter as an opportunity to extend discussion around a key theme that arose in the workshop which has not yet been specifically discussed in this book – that of *reflective practice* – and to consider some elements and practical strategies that support ongoing reflection in practice, as suggested by our participants. Reflective practice is certainly an element that underpins many of the initiatives and strategies discussed throughout this book, however it has not been explicitly defined and we feel that it deserves further discussion here.

In the same way that evidence-based practice (EBP) has become a buzzword, as discussed in Chapter 2, so reflective practice has also become a zeitgeist across the healthcare professions. Reflective practice was first described by Schön (1983) and this continues to be the seminal text, which we highly recommend to speech and language therapists (SLTs). Reflective practice has been defined as one of a range of critical thinking skills that help practitioners to be more explicit in their clinical reasoning and decision-making (Schön, 1983; Davies and van der Gaag, 1992). It also constitutes one of the core professional competencies that underpins SLT knowledge and skills (Royal College of Speech and Language Therapists, 2003).

Reflective practice can be encouraged through formal processes such as supervision or mentoring, or simply through individual clinicians taking time to reflect on their clinical decision making, knowledge, care processes and outcomes. This may include accessing and reading the research evidence base, reflecting on what has happened in therapy, and – as one of our workshop participants put it, thinking about 'what worked, what didn't'.

Without this reflection, it is easy to keep our heads down and continue to work as we always have – but thinking about what we are doing, why we are doing it, and whether or not it is working can be the basis for recognizing the shortfalls in our own knowledge and may suggest areas where we need to seek out more evidence to guide our practice. Some specific examples of actions that support reflection were suggested by our participants and are considered further below. These include establishing reading routines to regularly access and reflect on the evidence base, and using audit and outcome measurement to reflect on the processes and outcomes of practice.

Establishing a reading routine

One component of taking time for reflection may be establishing a reading routine in order to keep up with the literature in a clinical area. Laine and Weinberg (1999) suggested that keeping up-to-date with new literature involves 'both learning new information we never knew before and relearning what we once knew but have forgotten' (pp. 99–100). It is not just about identifying the latest assessment or therapy techniques, but is also about revising our understanding of the basics of our practice, keeping our skills and knowledge sharp. It is a reflective process because it involves comparing what we know and what we do (i.e. the techniques and approaches we are currently using) to those in the literature.

Most of us would agree that we regularly read professional literature, particularly the newsletters or magazines from our professional organizations. Peer-reviewed journals that we have on subscription are often scanned for papers that match our clinical interests before we set them aside. These are familiar reading habits for many of us. Yet a study examining new publications in primary care suggested that over 7000 new articles in healthcare (including new research, letters, editorials, and commentaries) are made available every month, and that doctors would need to set aside 627.5 hours per month to read these articles (Alper *et al.*, 2004). Obviously, the SLT literature base is significantly smaller than that of primary care, nevertheless, the number of new publications each month relevant to SLTs is likely to be beyond the capacity of individuals to identify, access, read and critically appraise.

Some strategies suggested in the literature for keeping up-to-date with current research, opinion and new knowledge and ideas are summarized below. It is worth noting that these suggestions come from the medical literature, but we feel that the suggestions may be useful for SLTs as well. We would emphasize that these approaches are just suggestions. Individual clinicians need to decide what will work best for them, and the strategies below may or may not resonate for you. It may be very helpful to talk with colleagues about how they have developed and maintained a regular routine.

Develop a personal goal for keeping up-to-date

Laine and Weinberg (1999) argued that individuals need to make a decision about what being 'current' means for them. This will include acknowledging that you, as an individual, cannot possibly read, appraise, digest and utilize all of the new knowledge that is available in your field. Laine and Weinberg suggested that individuals ask themselves 'what information must I carry around in my head in order to be satisfied with my fund of knowledge?' Consider the information that you need to do your specific job, for example, knowledge relevant to your specific patient populations, and the treatments you offer. Also take into consideration the questions that patients, families or students commonly ask you about your area, as well as information that you feel any SLT in your field should know. These steps may be useful to narrow down the scope of reading that you attempt to tackle (Laine and Weinberg, 1999).

Make an 'A list' of journals and other sources of up-to-date information

With little time available to read, making the most of it by going to the best sources is vital. In a seminal paper discussing how doctors access the medical literature, Haynes and colleagues (1986) suggested creating a personalized reading list that incorporates only the best, most likely sources of information for your work, and ignores 'low-yield' sources (i.e. sources that provide low quality articles or those that only now and then have articles relevant to you). Laine and Weinberg (1999) also highlight that 'filtering' is an essential part of keeping up-to-date. That is, choosing to spend precious reading time only on those sources that are likely to provide us with the information that we need. This includes taking into consideration the strength of the source in providing peer-reviewed, scientific literature which is of relevance to clinical practice. This doesn't mean that only journal articles are appropriate however, and Laine and Weinberg (1999) point out that a number of sources, including things like clinical practice guidelines, may be worth spending time reading, because they are essentially summaries of the latest evidence, and they have strong relevance for practice.

Become an efficient browser

As well as targeting your reading toward likely 'high yield' sources, becoming more efficient in browsing through tables of contents and abstracts can increase the amount that you are able to get through in your reading time. Cook *et al.* (1996) suggested that even browsing should be targeted towards those sources that are most likely to be relevant. For example, journal alerts can be set up for those sources that often provide articles relevant to your clinical practice.

Create summaries that you can easily refer to

Summarizing a paper is a good way to ensure that you have read it thoroughly enough to identify the key issues and clinical implications. Cook *et al.* (1996) suggest that creating a short critical summary of the article or of several articles around the one topic (i.e. creating a 'critically appraised topic' summary) can be a useful way to both organize and store new information from your reading time. The development of critically appraised papers and topics (CATs and CAPs) was discussed by Tracy, Rachel and Rachelle in Chapter 18, which includes an example template that could be used to create a CAP from your own reading. Summarizing a paper can also just include a quick 'bullet point' summary of the key points of the article, for example:

- key question addressed
- major findings
- clinical implications that are relevant to your practice
- reference information about the article (i.e. authors, journal, volume and page numbers, title of article)

Store information effectively so that you can refer to it again when needed

Having spent your time reading and reflecting, it is important that the key information that you identify is kept to refer to later. There is nothing more frustrating than searching blindly for that one paper that you remember reading a few months ago, which you realize is exactly what you now need. A systematic approach to filing and indexing articles and your notes from these is important. If you are already familiar with one of the software packages that indexes your references then you won't need any convincing to use it, although you still need to invest some thought and consistency into your own key terms, so that you will indeed be able to track down that elusive paper. Software is not essential, as paper index cards still work well for many people. For some people, simply sorting and filing digital or hard copies of papers or critical summaries under key words or topic headings that are relevant to you may be enough. If you are going to use a software system, be sure to talk to colleagues, as it's best to choose the one used and supported locally, so that you know where to go for assistance while you're getting familiar with using it, and so that you can easily share your references with your colleagues.

Evaluating practice: audit and outcome measurement

A formal way of approaching reflective practice is through audit and outcome measurement. Both of these evaluative processes allow SLTs to step back and to reflect, considering both the processes of care and the impact that these processes are having for individual patients. EBP has a focus on improving the processes of clinical care – what happens to a patient when they come to a SLT for diagnosis and/or treatment. In undertaking audit, SLTs assess whether they are in fact providing the care that the evidence (including patient preferences, clinical knowledge and published research) suggests they should be. Outcome measurement provides information about the effectiveness of evidence-based care. While assessment and treatment approaches may have good evidence for their *efficacy* (i.e. they have a demonstrated effect in controlled, research situations), outcome measurement allows clinicians to examine the *effectiveness* of care when evidence-based methods are applied to real clients in the clinical setting. The research evidence may suggest that treatment A is the most effective, but what has it done for this patient, in this situation? The focus for outcome measurement is on the patient (Butler, 1995) and it facilitates our understanding about what 'works' in the context of everyday clinical care, not just in the world of research.

Although there is not room in this chapter for an in-depth description of audit and outcome measurement procedures or tools for SLTs, we have summarized some of the key steps in each approach in the rest of this chapter.

Audit approaches

Box 33.1 summarizes the steps taken in an audit. It should be noted that audit approaches can be used for evaluating many components of what we do, but the emphasis in this chapter is on the use of audits in evaluating whether or not the processes of care reflect what is known from the evidence. For example, if we agree that a certain approach has the best evidence, is this approach being applied every time it should be?

Box 33.1   Steps taken in audit

* *Choose processes to be evaluated.* Clinical practice has hundreds of processes and it is impossible to evaluate them all in one go. Processes should be prioritized based on those that are most likely to impact on patient outcomes (Fraser *et al.*, 1997). For example, if the evidence indicates that the number of sessions is more important than the location of therapy, then audit should focus on the number of sessions that clients received compared to agreed standards.
* *Choose standards for these processes.* The standards against which processes are measured should be set based on the evidence, and on locally agreed policies and guidelines.
* *Collect data on these processes and compare against standards.* Data collection doesn't have to involve a long, drawn out process. The Institute for Healthcare Improvement (2009) suggests that, where possible, data should be: *simple* (e.g. making use of existing information systems or using a simple form that is straightforward for staff to complete within their daily routine), *sampled* (a well-chosen sample is better than attempting to collect data on everything), *targeted* (based on the processes and standards that you defined at the beginning).
* *Provide feedback about the results to SLTs.* Feedback about the results of audit is essential to promote change in practice (Jamtvedt *et al.*, 2006). Feedback should focus on the processes and standards prioritized at the beginning of the audit- for example, how many times are patients receiving the agreed number of sessions of therapy? Discussion around the results may yield some fruitful paths for further inquiry and/or improvement. For example, staff may identify barriers to providing the required number of sessions (e.g. patients failing to remember appointments) which may suggest a need to look at the evidence for the best ways to improve this (e.g. through paper or text message reminders).

The use of an audit approach has been demonstrated in this book by several authors, for example Angela (Chapter 22) evaluated the existing processes of assessment used in her paediatric stroke service. Having identified that these processes were unsystematic and lacking in a guiding framework, her team undertook to develop systematic protocols for SLT assessment of children post-stroke.

Outcome measurement

There are many forms of outcome measurement, but the general steps required are summarized in Box 33.2.

Box 33.2   Steps taken in outcome measurement

- *Choose appropriate measurement domains.* Outcome measurement should be based on the goals of therapy, and these goals are not the same in every clinical situation. For example, when working with young children with speech sound disorders, the goals of therapy may include:
    - that the child's ability to articulate certain speech sounds improves
    - that the child's overall intelligibility improves
    - that the child is able to participate more frequently at preschool
    - that the child's parents are able to effectively monitor and provide modelling and feedback to support their child's speech.
- *Chose an appropriate outcome measure.* There are many existing outcome measures for SLTs. In addition to taking into account the overall aims and specific goals of therapy, SLTs may need to consider the patient population in question, as some measures are disorder and/or age-specific.
- *Measure outcomes.* Routine outcome measurement may include evaluating patient function, quality of life, impairment, participation (and so on) before and after an episode of care. Measuring before and after care has taken place is important in order to measure change (e.g. improvement) or stability. Some outcome measures are only relevant at the end of therapy – for example, satisfaction with care.
- *Provide feedback to SLTs.* Like audit data, outcomes data is only valuable if it is used. As we evaluate the outcomes of clinical care in practice, outcome measurement data also contributes to the evidence base for the management of a disorder (Pring, 2004). Outcomes data may provide information to direct clinical decision-making as well as guide the direction of future clinical research. Kane (2006) argued that outcomes data 'should be seen as complementing, not competing, with RCTs' (p. 5). Enderby (1997) pointed out that outcome measurement should allow clinicians and managers 'to ask intelligent questions' about practice, which would guide formal research.

The range of outcome domains that may be relevant for SLTs to consider is broad, and may include (Enderby, 1992; Schunk, 1996; Cameron, 1997; Frattali, 1998; Hesketh and Hopcutt, 1997;): *clinical/ impairment outcomes* (e.g. changes in impairment related to the intervention); *functional outcomes* (the impact on an aspect of the patient's ability that has a real life meaning to the patient); *patient satisfaction* with care; *social outcomes* (e.g. level of employability, participation); *knowledge outcomes* (including patient or carer knowledge about the condition and its management); *quality of life and wellbeing outcomes;* and *indirect outcomes* (for example, discharge destination, amount of assistance required by family or carers).

The specific aim of therapy makes a difference to the way that outcomes are measured and evaluated- for example, if the aim is maintenance, then the outcome that should be measured is not whether someone has improved, but whether their skills, function, abilities, and so on, have been preserved over time. Malcomess

(2001) described eight possible 'aims' of speech and language therapy: assessment, anticipatory, curative, re/habilitative, maintenance, enabling, supportive, and palliative.

Outcome measurement has also been demonstrated in various ways throughout this book, for example Amanda and Leora (Chapter 27) measured health outcomes (e.g. acute illness, pneumonia), and Shalini (Chapter 20) evaluated the activities of children, the attitudes of the villagers towards the children, as well as changes in oral communication skills and student learning.

Summary

The workshop at the RCSLT conference provided us with an opportunity to extend our understanding of what 'embedding EBP' really means for SLTs. We have emphasized the theme of reflective practice in this chapter, as it is an important concept underpinning EBP. This section has demonstrated some approaches to embedding reflection through regular reading and through evaluating processes and outcomes of care. As Pam Enderby has challenged us all in her foreword to this book, we need to all become more reflective and critical reviewers of our own practice.

References

Alper, B.S., Hand, J.A., Elliott, S.G., *et al.* (2004) How much effort is needed to keep up with the literature relevant for primary care. *Journal of the Medical Library Association*, **92** (4), 429–437.

Butler, C. (1995) Outcomes that matter. *Developmental Medicine and Child Neurology*, **37**, 753–754.

Cameron, I. (1997) Measurement of outcomes in rehabilitation medicine. Paper presented at the Integrating Health Outcomes Measurement in Routine Health Care Conference, Canberra.

Cook, D.J., Meade, M.O. and Fink, M.P. (1996) How to keep up with the critical care literature and avoid being buried alive. *Critical Care Medicine*, **24** (10), 1757–1768.

Davies, P. and van der Gaag, A. (1992) The professional competence of speech therapists III: skills and skill mix possibilities. *Clinical Rehabilitation*, **6**, 311–323.

Enderby, P. (1992) Outcome measures in speech therapy: Impairment, disability, handicap and distress. *Health Trends*, **24** (2), 61–64.

Enderby, P. (1997) The art and science of measuring outcomes. *RCSLT Bulletin*, 7.

Fraser, R.C., Khunti, K., Baker, R. and Lakhani, M. (1997) Effective audit in general practice: a method for systematically developing audit protocols containing evidence-based review criteria. *British Journal of General Practice*, **47**, 743–746.

Frattali, C.M. (1998) Outcomes measurement: Definitions, dimensions, and perspectives. In C.M. Frattali (ed.), *Measuring Outcomes in Speech–Language Pathology*. New York: Thieme, (pp. 1–27).

Haynes, R.B., McKibbon, K.A., Fitzgerald, D., Guyatt, G.H., Walker, C.J. and Sackett, D.L. (1986) How to keep up with the medical literature: III. Expanding the number of journals you read regularly. *Annals of Internal Medicine*, **105** (3), 474–478.

Hesketh, A. and Hopcutt, B. (1997) Outcome measures for aphasia therapy: it's not what you do, it's the way that you measure it. *European Journal of Disorders of Communication*, **32** (3), 203–216.

Institute for Healthcare Improvement (2009) Tips for effective measures. *Journal.* Retrieved 12 October 2009 from http://www.ihi.org/IHI/Topics/Improvement/ ImprovementMethods/Measures/tipsforestablishingmeasures.htm

Jamtvedt, G., Young, J.M., Kirstoffersen, D.T., O'Brien, M.A. and Oxman, A.D. (2006) Audit and feedback: effects on professional practice and health care outcomes. *Cochrane Database of Systematic Reviews*, **2**, CD000259.

Kane, R.L. (2006) Introduction. In R.L. Kane (ed.), *Understanding Health Care Outcomes Research*. Boston: Jones and Bartlett, pp. 3–22.

Laine, C. and Weinberg, D.S. (1999) How can physicians keep up-to-date? *Annual Review of Medicine*, **50**, 99–110.

Malcomess, K. (2001) The reason for care. *RCSLT Bulletin*, 12–14.

Pring, T. (2004) Ask a silly question: two decades of troublesome trials. *International Journal of Language and Communication Disorders*, **39**, 285–302.

Royal College of Speech and Language Therapists (2003) Reference framework: Underpinning competence to practise. *Journal.* Retrieved 13 October 2009 from http:// www.rcslt.org/docs/competencies_project.pdf

Schön, D. (1983) *The Reflective Practitioner*. London: Basic Books.

Schunk, C. (1996) Outpatient outcomes: you can collect the data, but you have to know what to do with it. *Rehab Management*, April/May, 105–107.

34 Embedding EBP: future directions

Hazel Roddam and
Jemma Skeat

So having come to the end of the book, what are we hoping may follow on from this initiative? We have already referred to the challenge we faced in inviting only a relatively small number of contributors to feature in this book. We know of so many more SLT colleagues who are dedicated to embedding EBP in their own daily work who could also have shared their stories if space had allowed. And we have no doubts that many of our readers will also have their own experiences to draw upon. We have particularly valued the opportunity to glean insights into the wider range of workplace settings afforded by our world-wide contributors and feel that this is an element that will benefit us all greatly. The national socioeconomic and political contexts significantly influence the way in which we all work, and these elements will continue to impact on our professional practice. For this reason we would very much value future opportunities to learn how our colleagues world-wide are addressing these issues.

There is such a lot that we can all learn from looking over each other's shoulders, and this book is just a starting place. The world wide web presents an obvious opportunity for further sharing, with web-based repositories of good practice initiatives and case studies that would serve as a resource for SLTs as one possibility for the future. This could be something led by the professional associations in each country, or by universities, other organizations, or even just interested SLTs, who are able to take the lead to organize and update these repositories. Professional conferences (both SLT specific and multidisciplinary) provide another chance for us to communicate with one another about the things that we are doing to embed EBP. Such contributions would complement the more traditional research activity presented at conferences, and help to more effectively bridge the research–practice gap.

One area that would be particularly valuable to learn more about is the initiatives and strategies by which SLTs are engaging with their service users. This would include ways of helping individual clients to be more actively involved in planning and evaluating their own treatment, as well as innovative approaches to engaging clients in consultations for either planning or evaluating wider service initiatives.

We would like to take this opportunity to discuss how much we have in common with our colleagues across the other allied health professions. For many of us, our clinical work takes place with the context of a multi-disciplinary team. Within healthcare settings, these teams comprise doctors and nursing staff as well as a wide range of other therapists. In community settings SLTs work in inter-professional teams with other therapists as well as cross-agency teams with teachers and classroom assistant staff, educational psychologists, plus social services professionals. Our colleagues in physiotherapy, occupational therapy and other relevant therapy groups all face the same challenges as we do to embed EBP into their clinical practice. They share the same drivers in terms of professional practice standards for continuing education and EBP, as well as for engagement with service users. Like us, they also have an evidence base which is variable across clinical conditions and intervention approaches. There is much that we can all profit from engaging with other professionals in order to promote and support EBP to become embedded into our routine practice. We would highly recommend readers to consider opportunities for initiatives such as multi-professional journal clubs (looking at multi-professional evidence bases); the development of multi-professional critically appraised topics/ critically appraised papers, perhaps through a 'network' structure as described in Chapter 18; and the collaborative development of local evidence-based protocols and care pathways. As with SLT initiatives, sharing our successes in using these strategies and approaches across professionals is a must.

We would like to thank you for taking the time to read this book. We hope that you have enjoyed the stories of our contributors and have found our commentaries useful in suggesting further resources or highlighting particular points. It is our aspiration that this publication will help to generate some more dialogue across the profession and will prompt SLTs to share their own thoughts and experiences with colleagues. We look forward to watching the evidence base grow over the coming years. But more importantly, we look forward to seeing the research evidence have a greater impact on SLT clinical practice, as EBP becomes more firmly embedded as a fundamental element of our professional identity.

Index

Also available from Wiley

Ethics in Speech and Language Therapy
By Richard Body and Lindy McAllister
ISBN: 9780470058886

Speech and Language Therapy: Issues in professional practice
By Caroline Anderson and Anna van der Gaag
ISBN: 9781861564610

Evidence Based Practice in Speech Pathology
By Sheena Reilly, Jacinta Douglas and Jenni Oates
ISBN: 9781861563200